Dreadful

DISEASES AND

TERRIBLE

TREATMENTS

METRO BOOKS
New York

An Imprint of Sterling Publishing Co., Inc.
1166 Avenue of the Americas
New York, NY 10036

© 2017 by Quid Publishing

ISBN 978-1-4351-6471-0

For information about custom editions, special sales, and premium and
corporate purchases, please contact Sterling Special Sales at 800-805-5489
or specialsales@sterlingpublishing.com.

Manufactured in China

2 4 6 8 10 9 7 5 3 1

www.sterlingpublishing.com

Design by Lindsey Johns

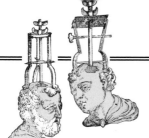

Dreadful
DISEASES AND
TERRIBLE
TREATMENTS

THE STORY OF MEDICINE THROUGH THE AGES

Jonathan J. Moore

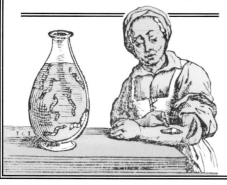

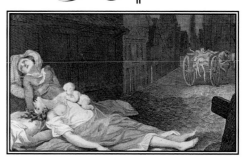

METRO BOOKS
NEW YORK

CONTENTS

Introduction 6

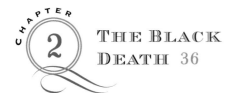

CHAPTER

1

COMMON
COMPLAINTS 12

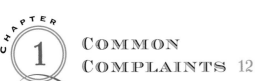

CHAPTER

2

THE BLACK
DEATH 36

CHAPTER

3

VENEREAL
DISEASE 64

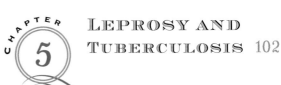

CHAPTER

4

SHOCKING
SURGERY 74

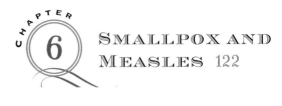

CHAPTER

5

LEPROSY AND
TUBERCULOSIS 102

CHAPTER

6

SMALLPOX AND
MEASLES 122

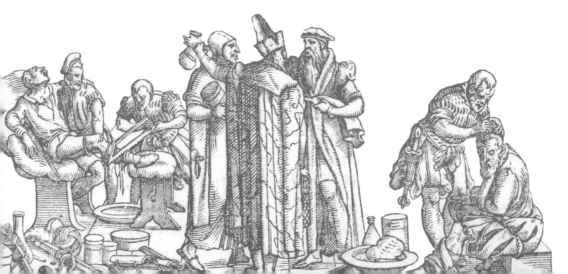

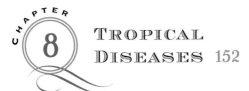 CHAPTER 7 TYPHUS FEVER 138

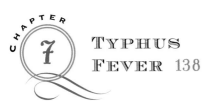 CHAPTER 8 TROPICAL DISEASES 152

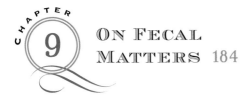 CHAPTER 9 ON FECAL MATTERS 184

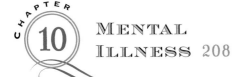 CHAPTER 10 MENTAL ILLNESS 208

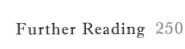 CHAPTER 11 SPANISH INFLUENZA 232

Further Reading 250

Index 252

Picture Credits 256

INTRODUCTION

THE CHANCES THAT WE ARE ALIVE ON PLANET EARTH ARE MILLIONS and billions or even trillions to one. So, enjoy every single second. There are 60 seconds in a minute, 60 minutes in an hour, 24 hours in a day, 365 days in a year, and 74 years in an expected lifetime. Therefore, you can expect to live for approximately two-and-a-quarter trillion seconds. There are 78 organs in the body and 12 major organ systems. Each body is composed of about 15 trillion cells that die and are replaced every 7 years. All of these organs and cells are vulnerable to 30,000 described diseases which attack the human body, two-thirds of which have no known cure.

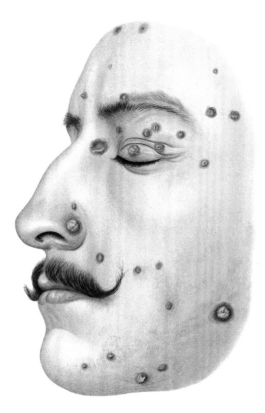

Chief among the threats to your life are an estimated 320,000 viruses. Viruses are a very common cause of infectious disease and many of the most common human ailments are viral.

Currently there are approximately 200 known viruses that cause disease in humans. Over 100 of these cause "colds." Viral diseases include: HIV/AIDS, the common cold, influenza, measles, rubella, chicken pox, mumps, polio, mononucleosis, Ebola, West Nile fever, chickenpox, smallpox, hepatitis, meningitis,

LEFT **Syphilis is caused by bacteria that infect a new host through sexual activity. It moves through three stages. Depicted here is the tertiary stage, with pustules breaking out all over the body.**

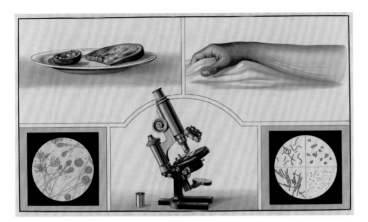

LEFT **By the 18th and 19th centuries the invention of effective microscopes led to the development of germ theory. Our understanding of illness moved from superstition to scientific observation.**

encephalitis, pneumonia, and SARS. Many viruses are hard to destroy without damaging or killing the living cells they infect; this is why drugs are often not used to control them. Many viral diseases can be prevented by immunization.

It is estimated that 500 to 1,000 species of bacteria live in the human gut. Bacterial cells are much smaller than human cells, and there are at least 10 times as many bacteria as human cells in the body. It is when these relatively harmless bacteria are allowed to thrive due to a weakened immune system, or move to a part of the body where they are not meant to be, that some of the worst illnesses occur.

Bacteria have the richest evolutionary history of all life on earth. The earth is about 4.5 billion years old; the oldest fossils are 1 billion years younger and they are primitive bacteria. They represent the earliest life forms, which probably evolved in the hot, primordial oceans or near hot, submerged springs. They have had a lot of time to evolve and learn how to survive in all kinds of environments. If bacteria attack humans, they are hard to get rid of. Arrayed against these ancient bugs and diseases are our frail immune systems.

BIOLOGICAL WARFARE

When a person gets ill, it often means that microbes (which include both viruses and bacteria) are trying to survive and reproduce, at our expense! The symptoms of an illness force us to miss work or even, in a worst-case scenario, kill us.

Microbes have evolved many diverse ways of spreading and ensuring the survival of their species. Some microbes hang around passively waiting to be ingested; examples are some worm infections and salmonella. Once ingested they replicate furiously, before passing through waste matter back into the environment, where they wait in soil or on plant matter until another host consumes them.

Others play havoc with their host's immune system, causing them to sneeze and cough, thus launching millions of their progeny into the atmosphere where they are inhaled or otherwise ingested into a new host in which they can continue breeding. Influenza, the common cold, and the more deadly whooping cough are examples of these transmission strategies. While these rather nasty diseases are transmitted through the respiratory tract, others are transmitted through the digestive tract. Cholera replicates at such a furious rate that sufferers void through their bowels up to 3 gallons (12 liters) of liquid "rice water" feces a day, thus infecting water sources with billions of bacteria waiting to be taken up by any poor soul who drinks the water.

Other microbes modify the anatomy or habits of their host to accelerate their transmission. Genital warts, syphilis, and smallpox cause sores to break out on the skin. Once another individual touches these infected points with their genitalia or any other body cavity or sore, the disease has a new invasion point. Rabies is a particularly nasty disease that gets into the saliva of an infected host and drives victims into a frenzy. Saliva foams out of their mouths and they attack and bite anything they see.

Blood-borne microorganisms such as those that cause typhus, malaria, and yellow fever, as well as a host of "microfilariae" (tiny worm-like creatures) repro-

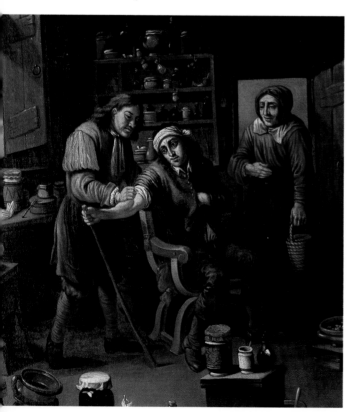

duce in the lymphatic system or the bloodstream so that they overwhelm the body's natural defenses and lead to multiple organ failure. Their huge numbers of offspring ensure that uninfected parasites or carriers such as lice and mosquitoes will pick them up in their feeding strategies and carry them to another host, where the process can begin again. Often these diseases can live and reproduce inside a host for decades. Malaria, carried by the *Anopheles* mosquito, hides in its host's kidneys, causing no symptoms until it emerges in random episodes into the bloodstream,

LEFT **Early remedies were usually based on traditional therapies and rarely cured the patient's condition. Here, a surgeon bleeds his patient.**

where the chances are that another mosquito will pick it up. Meanwhile, the poor human carrier has to endure agonizing pain, fevers, and delirium. The disease then vacates the bloodstream and hibernates in the liver until the next attack.

Other more deadly diseases employ all of these strategies and more. The bubonic plague may begin as bacteria dormant in dried rodent feces. Once inhaled, it can then move into the lymphatic system, leading to buboes that burst under the pressure of infectious pus. Or else it migrates directly into the bloodstream where biting fleas pick it up and transmit it into other hosts. The bacteria can then penetrate the lung walls, becoming pneumonic plague, which is transmitted through coughing and sneezing, leading to a 98 percent mortality rate in a matter of hours. Ebola is a more recently discovered disease with a similar life cycle. It can be passed on through even the smallest contact through semen, saliva, blood, flesh, or mucus.

The law of infection is simple: As long as a microbe—virus, bacterium, protozoan, or worm—infects one new victim before its original host dies, it will survive. If it can infect a hundred, a thousand, or a million new carriers, that's even better.

From Hunter–Gatherer to Metropolis

Bones from ancient nomadic peoples display few signs of disease. Fractures, breaks, blunt force trauma, and rheumatism are as common as lost limbs, but evidence of infectious disease is rarely found.

Hunter–gatherer societies living in diverse isolated locations were not prey to constant recurrences of epidemic diseases. They suffered from heritage diseases, which may have existed in our ancestors' populations well before they emerged from the treetops to become upright hominids. Characteristic of these diseases is that they take a long time to kill their hosts and indeed may not kill them at all, attaining a kind of symbiosis where disease and host coexist. Some heritage diseases, such as hemophilia, are genetic in nature and only strike selected populations.

Other infections of small human populations are chronic diseases that take a long time to kill the victims, allowing them to linger alive and act as a reservoir of microbes to infect other members of the tribe. Yaws, leprosy, and tuberculosis are characteristic of these infections, as are many types of parasitic infections such as worms.

The mobility of hunter–gatherer tribes protected them to an extent, as they were able to leave behind infested areas, and this may have caused the pathogen to die out or reduce its virulence. Highly contagious members of the tribe were left behind if the infection overwhelmed their immune system, preventing further infection within the group.

House-Proud Neanderthals

There is some evidence that the cave-dwelling populations of Neanderthal Man made an effort to keep their caves clean. Shelters were divided into different occupation zones that maximized hygiene. Rather than just tossing carcasses anywhere to rot and be scavenged, there were separate food preparation and butchering areas, cooking areas, and living areas where food was consumed. Tools were stored in one section of the cave and there was a workshop at the mouth of the cave where the light was best.

The middle regions of caves appear to have been the main living and sleeping areas and contain the most traces of human occupation. Sections of the caves farthest away from the entrance appear to have been used as a storage area to reduce clutter around the hearth. Animal bones and stone tools were concentrated at the front rather than the rear of the shelter. These highly organized living spaces show a degree of commonality over many Neanderthal sites, indicating that managing waste and promoting basic hygiene was practiced by all Neanderthal populations.

Once humans settled in permanent agricultural communities they exposed themselves to a new host of infectious pathogens. These are usually termed "crowd diseases." Farmers are sedentary and live among their own sewage and the waste from any domesticated species. These concentrated populations allowed microbes to thrive and gave them a short path from one person's body into another's drinking water or lungs. Cholera and influenza are among the classic crowd diseases.

Early settlements might become death traps. Farmers used their own waste as fertilizer, spreading their parasites to all of their neighbors. Rats moved in to feast on the farmers' produce, leaving waste and disease in their wake. Irrigation allowed schistosomiasis parasites (causing blindness and elephantiasis) to thrive, along with mosquitoes and all of the deadly infections they carry to infect millions of humans. Farmers took it one step further. By domesticating animals they allowed hundreds of diseases, such as tuberculosis and rabies, to cross the species barrier causing previously unheard-of ailments.

As cities became larger, a constant trend of migration from the rural poor led to a never-ending supply of new hosts; this uninterrupted population resource allowed microbes to thrive and mutate for maximum effect. The collapse of Western civilization after the Roman Empire can be put down to lethal crowd diseases. Once the European population had dispersed through the Dark Ages, there were fewer incidents of crowd diseases racing through the population.

With the increase in populations through the Middle Ages, the Renaissance, and into modern times, a new golden age of crowd diseases emerged. Nasty bugs such as cholera, typhoid, influenza, tuberculosis, yellow fever, smallpox, and measles had unprecedented access to fertile pastures where they could—and still do—harvest millions of people every year.

Crowd diseases were most lethal where colonial powers brought them into populations that had not had any opportunity to develop resistance or an immune response. Beginning with the conquistadors, populations throughout the New World and the Pacific were decimated as virgin populations were almost destroyed by microscopic foreign invaders. Modern medicine has alleviated some of the risks but disease remains a clear and present danger.

DREADFUL DISEASES AND TERRIBLE TREATMENTS

This book can't hope to cover all of the dreadful diseases that have infected humans throughout history, but it does try to shine a light on some of the worst infections and their effect on humankind. It also covers some of the ways in which we puny humans have tried to keep mortality at bay through medicine and surgery—some methods having more success than others.

Over hundreds of generations hunter–gatherer societies built up the knowledge of how to set bones and use herbal remedies. Nevertheless, they also turned to superstition and magic in the hope of curing mysterious ailments. The ancient Greeks and Romans tried to establish logic-based cures, and many sound medical advances and diagnoses were made during this era. However, most of this knowledge was lost with the collapse of the Roman Empire. It was only during the Renaissance that the first modern medical practices, such as the use of ligatures in amputations, began to develop. This was partly as a result of dissection being made legal, allowing medics to gain a deeper understanding of how the human body works. Yet it was only with the dawn of modern technology in the 18th and 19th centuries that sound scientific-based medical practices, such as inoculations and the sterilization of medical instruments, began to replace traditional folk cures, which often did more harm than good. This book traces some of these developments and catalogs some of the very worst ill-advised treatments trialed in history.

RIGHT **The widespread use of vaccination in the 19th and 20th centuries saw the demise of one of man's deadliest enemies: smallpox.**

1

COMMON COMPLAINTS

UNTIL THE 19TH CENTURY, CURES WERE OFTEN BASED ON SUPERSTITION and guesswork. Many of them bore little correlation to the conditions they sought to remedy. From applying leeches to administering fecal-based medicines, doctors used a whole host of unlikely remedies to treat common complaints such as colds, headaches, and tooth decay, as well as more serious conditions such as gout, epilepsy, and scurvy.

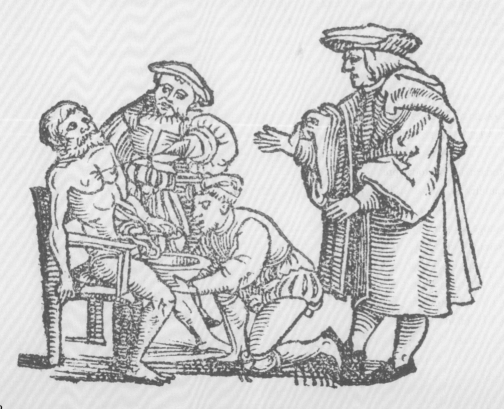

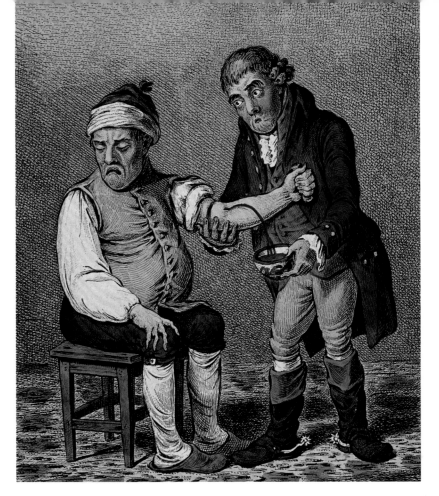

LANCETS AND LEECHES: THE ANCIENT CURE-ALL

ABOVE The bleeding of patients was a panacea in the medieval and early modern period. The practice often did more harm than good.

Modern doctors today prescribe bloodletting for those suffering from hemochromatosis (inherited iron overload disorder). This rare genetic disorder leads to iron accumulating in the bloodstream and can produce a range of symptoms including diabetes and liver collapse. A simple treatment of draining some blood can fix the problem.

Unfortunately for countless patients in the medieval period, extracting blood was seen as a cure-all for every type of illness, despite the fact that it was often the last nail in the coffin for many ailing individuals. Dropsy, the vapors, broken limbs, hysteria, consumption, and gout—any and every ailment was treated with bloodletting. Bloodletting was not only seen as a cure, it was also treated as a kind of spring-cleaning for the body. Just as we might take aspirin today, in the 17th and 18th centuries the well-to-do were cut and bled.

The most common form of bloodletting involved a nick with a sharpened (but not cleaned) lancet into a vein, usually near the inner elbow. Spring knives (held against the skin and containing a sharp blade which was triggered by the user) were also common; these handy devices allowed patients to bleed themselves and became a must-have for many gentlemen.

These little procedures could go awry; Queen Caroline of Bavaria (1792–1873) didn't just get a little nick on her forearm but bled to death after her artery was cut.

The bloodsucking leech was so commonly used that doctors were known as "leeches"—"to leech" meant "to cure." Recorded from 900 CE, leeches are still used today in certain circumstances.

Any good surgeon or barber would have a "ganon" (meaning group) of leeches. The most commonly used was *Hirudo medicinalis* (European medicinal leech), a creature about 1½ inches (4 cm) long that expands to as much as 6 inches (15 cm) once engorged. These creatures are perfectly designed for their purpose: They have suckers at both ends of their body and a total of 20 stomachs. Stored in a jar, they would be taken out an hour before use to work up an appetite. Placed in a glass or deposited with tweezers on the victim, it took 15 minutes for them to eat their fill, whereupon they would drop off their host. Alternatively, if short of leeches, the surgeon could snip off the tail of his leech, which would then keep drinking, a sort of bottomless pump.

Leeching was big business. In 1822 alone, London doctors imported 7 million leeches from Bordeaux (France) and Lisbon (Portugal). The English physician John Coakley Lettsom (1744–1815) required a daily relay of six horses to service the 82,000 calls he made during a calendar year.

TOP RIGHT **A scarificator with six lancets. This tool allowed the surgeon to make small incisions, thus reducing scarring.**

LEFT **Leeches were used to bleed patients. Anticoagulants contained in the leech's saliva may have had some minimal benefit.**

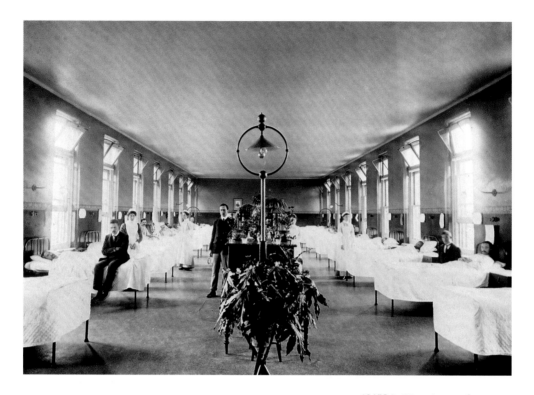

BED REST

Nurses as well as doctors have been responsible for using methods which are detrimental to a patient's health. An example of this was the commonly prescribed cure of bed rest. This can be appropriate for short-term illnesses that require rest while a nasty bug or virus is conquered by the body's defensive mechanisms, but in the past nurses and doctors often enforced long-term bed rest that was detrimental to patients. It was once assumed that bed rest had some magical healing property so that patients could devote all of their strength to healing. Autocratic head nurses often liked to ensure that their patients were wrapped up as tightly as possible, so that any movement was well-nigh impossible. This ensured a quiet and neat ward, something greatly admired in hospitals of the Victorian era (1837–1901) and the early 20th century.

One problem: Prolonged rest can be harmful. Patients who have been confined for a month will take at least the same time to build up their health afterward. The body responds to the demand placed upon it, and if no physical activity is practiced there will be a notable decline in fitness. Muscles atrophy, bones lose density and weaken, joints stiffen and become restricted in their movement, the heart loses

King Charles II

Charles II of England (lived 1630–85) was an unfortunate fellow. As the king lay on his deathbed, his 12 surgeons tried every "modern" technique in their arsenal to cure him. He was bled, purged, cupped, given sneezing powder, laxatives, emetics, absinthe, bitter water, and thistle leaves. The royal feet were smeared with pigeon excrement. None of these "cures" worked and he continued to decline. In a last desperate bid to revive him, 40 drops of extract from a man's skull were administered—all to no avail, and the king passed away. Without his doctors' help, Charles might have lived until 1700!

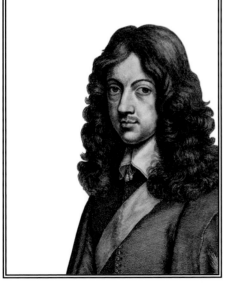

efficiency, deep vein thrombosis occurs along with osteoporosis and, in a worst-case scenario, blood clots can form and cause pulmonary embolism and death. Older people in particular were often made to undergo bed rest, and this led to many having drastically reduced life spans. Modern hospitals know now that untidy wards are good wards if patients are up and about using their bodies.

WASTE NOT, WANT NOT

Feces and urine were often used as a medicine during the Renaissance period (14th to 17th centuries). Dried, ground, smoked, distilled, or fermented, human waste could be mixed with a wide range of ingredients to be applied as a poultice, drunk as a medicine, or smeared on the skin.

That patients could live with the smell of human feces or the taste of fermented urine in their mouths gives an indication of the level of filth reached by European society at this time. While these cures might seem crazy to us now, at the time human waste and blood were seen as surefire remedies.

Farmers still use human waste as a fertilizer, and fullers (cloth finishers), laundrymen, and dyers have utilized fermented urine as a cheap source of ammonia, which is used to whiten cloth. So valuable was animal dung that it was often left in people's wills to a worthy beneficiary.

It was also used as a cure. Ancient Romans treated rashes in the diaper area by rubbing on a mixture of old urine with burnt oyster shells. In the West Highlands of Scotland it was advised to dry and powder human excrement and blow it in the eye to cure blindness. The dung of an infant was seen as particularly effective. Two teaspoons of the same taken daily was thought to cure epilepsy.

Distilled oil from the feces of children was thought to be an effective cure for dandruff when applied to the scalp. Distillation is a smelly business at best, but distilling feces must have been a particularly horrible activity. The same oil taken orally was considered a cure for cancer in 13th-century France. If urine was "stale and rank" it could be drunk to cure pleurisy, fever, and asthma, while constipation was tackled by a stiff draught of one's own urine every morning followed by one or two hours of fasting.

Barbecued dog feces strapped to a wound was recommended by the countess of Kent in the 17th century. Distilled horse, chicken, ox, and pig feces were prescribed for pleurisy. A jaundiced patient could be cured if he or she urinated on warm, steaming horse dung. Peacock dung cured vertigo. Rat droppings, five a day, were a cure for constipation. A balding fellow who wanted to make himself more appealing to the opposite sex was advised to mix rat droppings with honey and onion, and smear the stuff onto his scalp to make the hair grow back and impress the ladies! Smegma, the white smelly dirt that gathers under a man's foreskin, was said to be a useful salve against bites such as scorpion stings.

ABOVE Many early toilets were designed not to get rid of human waste, but rather to collect it for medicinal use.

Medical practitioners of this period swore by another unusual cure for a number of maladies. The urine of a 12-year-old boy would be left to ferment for several months before being mixed with a variety of herbs. It would then be administered orally. Apothecaries believed in the efficiency of this remedy and reported that few patients returned with further complaints, or for a second dose—this is not surprising! Equally efficient was the recipe calling for 2 drams of dried and powdered infant dung, which, if taken for several days, would cure epilepsy. How many repeat prescriptions of these wonder cures would be filled today, I wonder!

A BALDING FELLOW WHO WANTED TO MAKE HIMSELF MORE APPEALING TO THE OPPOSITE SEX WAS ADVISED TO MIX RAT DROPPINGS WITH HONEY AND ONION, AND SMEAR THE STUFF ONTO HIS SCALP TO MAKE THE HAIR GROW BACK.

Fair of Feces

Human waste was also used in cosmetics. Women in ancient Rome smeared feces over their faces to preserve a youthful complexion. In Restoration England (1660–85), women washed their faces in their own urine, and ashes of goats' dung mixed with oil stopped them losing their hair. To clear the pores, they washed their faces with honey, vinegar, milk, and a boy's urine.

Countess Elizabeth Báthory of Hungary (1560–1614) retained her youthful looks by bathing in virgins' blood, but in the late 18th century a French noblewoman discovered her own elixir of youth, as reported by the respected physician M. Geoffroy. She retained a fine, strapping young male servant whose sole function within the household was to defecate into a tin-plated copper pot with a tight lid. Once the stool had cooled, he was to carefully lift the lid and scrape condensed moisture from its surface into a flask, from which the woman anointed her cheeks and hands every evening and so retained her girlish complexion.

LEFT **Legend has it that Elizabeth Báthory of Hungary bathed in the blood of freshly killed virgin peasant girls.**

BLOOD AND BODY PARTS

Epilepsy, or the "falling sickness," was a catchall in Europe that covered a range of complaints including those we now term stroke, heart attack, low blood pressure, and, of course, epilepsy. Human body parts and in particular human blood were seen as particularly good at curing these conditions.

In Renaissance Europe it was believed that drinking human blood could cure all types of ailments including congestion, epilepsy, painful menstruation, and even flatulence. The younger the blood, the more potent the cure, so the blood of recently executed young men was seen as most effective, as it was possessed of the most vigor. Sufferers of these conditions paid generously to buy warm blood.

Blood was collected in handkerchiefs, cups, and jugs. Often the person who consumed the blood would run away from the scene of the execution at top speed. These strange behaviors reveal the reasoning behind these cannibalistic practices. It was believed that such a strong charge of youthful vitality could lead to intemperate and violent behavior, so it was necessary to exhaust the body to enable the medicine to do its work without catastrophic side effects. Similarly, the still warm blood was seen as being so beneficial that it was important to spread it throughout the body as quickly as possible, and the best way to do this was to engage in physical activity. This superstition lasted until quite recent times in Germany, with the last recorded incident in Berlin in 1864. Best of all was to drink the blood of a red-headed young man, as they were believed to be the most energetic of all!

There were other variations. Cats' blood was seen as beneficial in some cases, and dipping the bloody executioner's sword in wine before drinking the wine was an appropriate substitute.

Not only blood was used. Cadavers from those who had died violently supplied a veritable cornucopia of products for medicinal usage in medieval and Renaissance Europe. Hair, saliva, liver, urine, earwax, feces, and the heart were all harvested from corpses and mixed up into a range of frightful unguents, ointments, and medicines.

A recipe produced in 1672 by Edward Bolnest gives an example of one typical medicinal ingredient. About 4 pounds (2 kg) of flesh taken from the thighs of a strong young man executed in the middle of August should be put in a jar and covered with alcohol for four days. It should then be placed on a glass, covered with salt, and left to cure outdoors until thoroughly dried. It could then be stored until small shavings or powder were required for use in medicines.

BELOW The skull was seen as the repository of a human's divine energy. Ground-up skull was often used in medicines.

Expensive cures for epilepsy utilized only the best ingredients. One required ground skull, gold, pearl, amber, coral, bezoar (a rocklike substance that forms in the gut of certain animals from compressed hair), and peony seed to be mixed together to form a tonic. It should then be mixed with herbal tea and administered seven days in a row. If the patient is male, a female skull is required in the recipe, and if the patient is female, the skull should come from a male. This fantastic array of ingredients was to ensure that the patient got value for money, even if it didn't work.

Dried human heart was another cure for epilepsy, as was a brew made from water of lily, malmsey, lavender, and 3½ pounds (1.5 kg) of human brain.

THE CRAZIEST CURES

HERE ARE SOME OF THE craziest random cures recorded in the annals of history:

- If a woman wanted to get pregnant, it was recommended that she drink horse semen.
- Wearing wolf pelts could cure skin cancer.
- A potent contraception was to wrap herbs in a linen scarf before wrapping it around your neck.
- It was believed that whooping cough could be cured by drinking water from the skull of a bishop. In Ireland, sheep droppings boiled in milk was a recipe used to treat whooping cough. If this did not work, it was recommended to carry the patient over and under a donkey nine times.
- If a woman had been in labor too long, the family was advised to run around the house banging doors and chest lids to facilitate the birth.
- A cure for warts was to touch the coat of a man who had never seen his father.
- Eating the beating heart of a swallow was believed to confer intelligence and improve the memory.
- The blood of a hare killed in March was good for skin inflammation.
- Fennel boiled with pigeon's blood could restore eyesight, as could hen blood boiled with human breast milk.
- A cure for cataracts was to apply the marrow of goose wing or the ashes of a burnt snail mixed in with dried human excrement, dry it, and blow it into the eye.
- Consuming burned female mule hoof combined with ashes was effective at preventing conception.
- An ingestion of powdered bladder or kidney stones fixed sore eyes.
- A cure for epilepsy was to roast an ass liver in the blood of a weasel, before mixing it with stones found in the belly of a sparrow. The mixture was placed in an amulet of buckskin and worn around the neck.
- John of Gaddesden (1280–1361), who was responsible for the health of King Edward II of England (1284–1327), would give those suffering from gallstones ground-up beetles, while those suffering from a poor spleen would have to consume the heads of seven fat bats.
- Warts could be healed by touching each growth with a separate pebble. The pebbles were then to be placed within a small leather bag, which was to be dropped on a path on the way to church. Whoever found the bag would start sprouting your warts.
- Mumps could be healed in the following manner: "Take a halter from an ass and place it around the patient's head. Then use it drag him around a pigsty three times."
- A bag full of cooked potatoes hung around the neck could cure the common cold. Or else rub a roast potato into the scalp.

Sir Kenelm Digby (1603–65), a much-respected natural philosopher, suggested grinding the skull of a violently killed man together with 2 ounces (60 g) of toenails or fingernails and dried mistletoe as a cure for the "falling sickness." Menstrual blood rubbed on the feet of epileptics was seen as an efficient method of preventing seizures.

One of the most ambitious recipes was provided by the German chemist Johann Schröder in his book *Zoologia* (1659). He needed a particularly fresh corpse, killed violently, to make his "divine water." First, the corpse complete with bowels, flesh, and bone had to be chopped up into very small pieces and pulverized until it was a large amorphous mass. The cadaver was then distilled and converted into a rich liquid. All a patient had to do was mix this confection with some of their own blood before downing the combination to cure any disease.

ABOVE **Johann Schröder (1600–64) advocated the use of human body parts in medicine.**

DENTAL CARE

Teeth recovered from early hominids and our hunter–gatherer ancestors rarely display tooth decay. A healthy diet based on naturally found fruits, nuts, and grains combined with meat from hunted animals ensured healthy teeth.

This changed in the Neolithic Period (10,000–2000 BCE), when farming techniques began to develop and humans lived in more settled societies. Just as crowd diseases took hold, so did decay. Production of grain meant more carbohydrates which meant more tooth decay.

The first reference to tooth decay comes from the Sumerians, who refer to "tooth worms" in documents from approximately 5000 BCE. It continued to be a problem in ancient societies and in 2600 BCE there is the first reference to a dental practitioner when the Egyptian Hesy-re's tomb inscription refers to him as "the greatest of those who deal with teeth."

By 500 BCE knowledge of teeth and their treatment had improved exponentially and writers in Greece, including Hippocrates (ca. 460–370 BCE) and Aristotle (384–322 BCE), are able to write about decay, gum disease, extraction with forceps, and the use of wires to stabilize loose teeth.

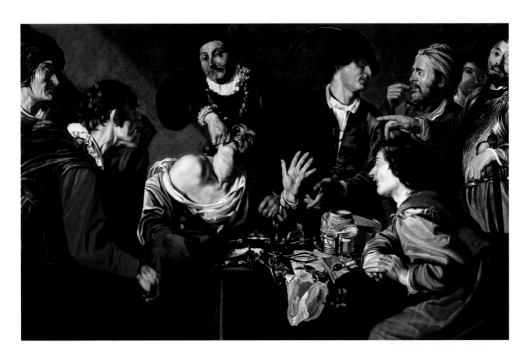

ABOVE Seventeenth-century barbers would often perform tooth extractions and bleed patients. Sometimes they traveled with theater troupes as part of the act.

The Etruscans in Italy (700–150 BCE) pioneered the use of dental prosthetics using gold crowns and fixed bridgework. (Even older Egyptian mummies have been found with false teeth but this appears have been done by embalmers after death.) In 700 CE the Chinese pioneered the use of a silver amalgam to fill cavities, a method which is only now being superseded.

In Europe, at the beginning of the 13th century, dental practitioners were formally recognized when the Guild of Barbers was established in France. These barbers were allowed to perform surgery, shaving, bleeding, tooth extraction, and, of course, haircuts. These practitioners often advertised their trade by wearing a necklace made up of all the rotten teeth they had extracted.

BELOW The Etruscans of Italy used dentures such as these as early as 700 BCE.

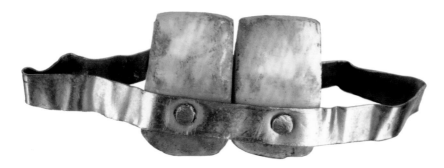

Tooth Decay

The Sumerian belief in tooth worms causing decay persisted right up until the 19th century. Egyptians, Indians, and the Chinese all believed in this nasty little character and the first European reference to the idea was in the 9th century CE.

Various methods were tried to get rid of tooth worms, including smoking them out or suffocating them with beeswax. Most often the tooth was extracted—painfully, without anesthetics.

Medieval Europeans had a wide range of methods to cure toothache. They included the following:

• Animal sperm was mixed with opium to kill pain or rubbed on the gums to cure toothache.

• To cure a toothache one had to write on paper "Jesus Christ for mercy's sake take away this toothache." The sufferer had to read it out aloud three times before burning the paper.

• Cavities could be filled with brain of partridge or crow dung, and it was recommended to bathe a tooth in bitch milk before extracting it.

• You could cure a sore tooth by touching it with one taken from an executed man.

This superstitious treatment of tooth decay only came to an end with the writings of Pierre Fauchard (1678–1761). Known as the father of modern dentistry, he made the link between sugar consumption and tooth decay.

At the same time as Fauchard was practicing, new inventions made it easier to extract teeth. One of the first of these was the "tooth key." It was the first specialized instrument to extract teeth and involved a claw that was placed over the tooth and a long bolster (metal rod) placed against the root. A quick twist and the whole tooth popped out. That was the theory, anyway. Often the roots stayed behind and had to be cut out individually.

BELOW **The taste for sugar in early modern Europe led to an epidemic of tooth decay. This 17th-century manuscript illustrates the range of forms rotting teeth took.**

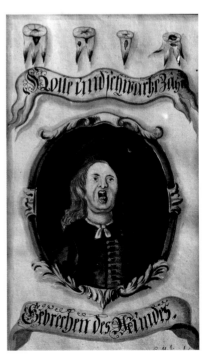

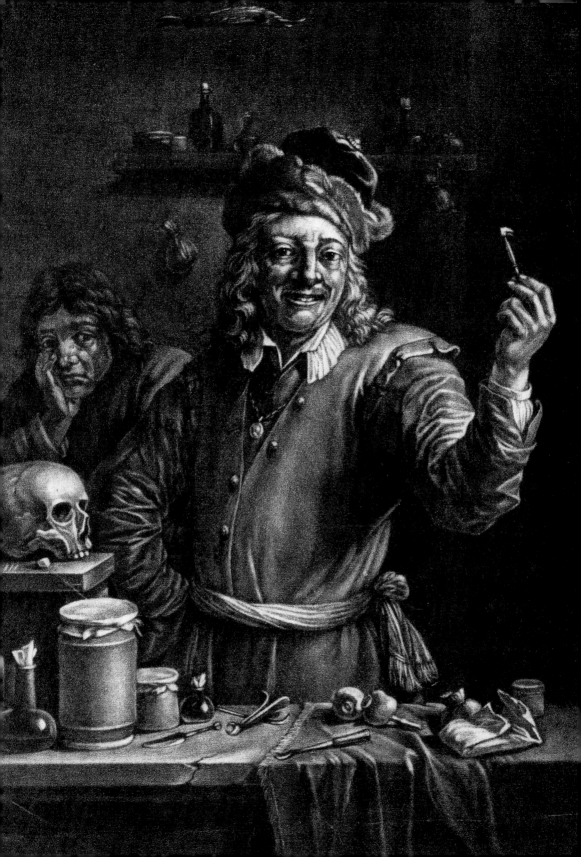

Implants and Falsies

One of the leading causes of premature death before the invention of penicillin was infected, pus-filled abscesses within the gums below infected teeth. A significant proportion of excavated skeletons reveal that these sores ate their way into the bone of upper and lower jaws. These often show no sign of healing, indicating that the wounds turned septic and killed the sufferer.

With the introduction of sugar into Europe after the colonization of the New World (1500) this problem became even worse. Mass tooth extractions were the order of the day, and those who retained their teeth often had mouths filled with blackened teeth that exhaled the stench of decay. Queen Elizabeth I of England (1533–1603) suffered from this complaint, and she was known not only for her red hair, but also for the fetid state of her teeth. Fashionistas of the Elizabethan period (1558–1603) artificially blackened their teeth with cosmetics.

Of course, with teeth being ripped out of swollen gums *en masse* it was necessary to replace them. Those of modest means would purchase wooden teeth, while wealthier individuals were able to obtain real teeth from corpses or donors.

Georgian England (1740–1830) saw the height of live tooth transplants. Sugar became cheap and plentiful, making it a part of every fashionable person's diet. Chefs competed with each other to create the most lavish sugar fancies. Tooth decay was rampant in the upper classes; young ladies sought transplants to replace their rotted teeth. One unscrupulous operator who took advantage of this was James Spence (and sons) operating out of the vice-ridden

LEFT **This early barber-surgeon looks pleased with himself. Not so his patient, who has just had a tooth drawn without the benefit of anesthetic.**

BELOW **In this 1787 etching, healthy teeth are extracted from a street urchin and implanted into the mouths of fashionable ladies.**

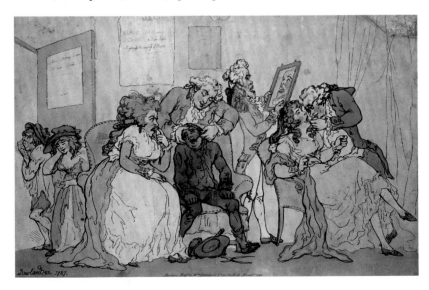

Soho district of London. Young women flocked to the Spence premises, determined to replace their teeth. Spence would send out his sons and assistants to trawl the local alleyways for young women who could donate their teeth. Suitable donors would then wait in one of his rooms while the customer waited in the adjacent operating room. Years of experience had given him great skills and Spence rapidly extracted teeth from the donors, gave them a cursory wipe to remove the blood, removed the rotted tooth from the patient, and jammed the new tooth into the swollen gums. The tooth was then secured in the jaw with twine tied to the adjacent teeth. The process was repeated until the young ladies could hold their heads high in society again.

Of course this was a perfect recipe for infection. Non-sterile tools and bacteria-laden teeth pushed into a bloody, already infected gum led to massive complications and, no doubt after a brief honeymoon, the patients learned to regret their decision. But worse was to come. Even after the transplanted teeth broke or fell out, syphilis (see pages 65–67) could appear, tiny bacteria on the tooth leading to corruption and huge rotting abscesses all around the jaw. At least seven of Spence's customers were infected. It was the advent of false ceramic teeth, or prosthetics using teeth from condemned criminals, that eventually closed him down.

As the middle classes continued to grow throughout Europe, so did the demand for realistic false teeth. The mother lode for teeth occurred after the Battle of Waterloo (June 1815). So many men died on the few square miles of this battlefield that hundreds of thousands of teeth were recovered from the corpses. These supplied the needs of British and French society with a good set of teeth for years. Local peasants roamed

BELOW A French dentist shows a potential customer the latest fashion in ceramic false teeth. They pass the closest scrutiny.

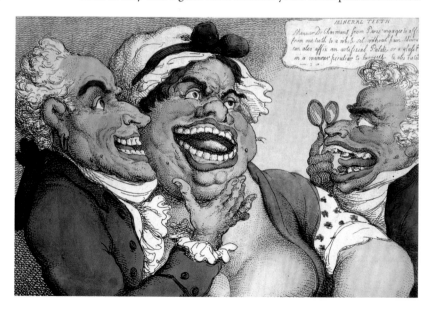

Nasty Inventions

Nothing strikes fear into people like the sound of a dental drill whirling away or the sight of a dentist's chair waiting for its next victim!

These fearsome inventions were created around 1790 by two Americans. John Greenwood adapted his mother's treadle spinning wheel to rotate the first dental drill. It was foot-powered and was called the "dental foot engine." Josiah Flagg invented the first dentist's chair by attaching an adjustable headrest and an arm extension to hold instruments to a wooden Windsor chair.

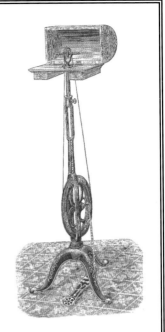

RIGHT **An early American dental drill. This cutting-edge technology utilized the foot pedal from a sewing machine.**

the field in the days after the battle, plundering clothes, shoes, and teeth. Tied together with gold or individually implanted, these teeth served their new owners for years after their original owners had rotted away in the mass graves around the battlefield. This practice continued late into the 19th century and even during the American Civil War (1861–65) professional tooth gatherers followed the armies and plundered the dead of their teeth. Such was the demand that during the 19th century a good set of teeth could fetch as much as five guineas.

Battlefields were not the only source of teeth. "Resurrectionists" (body snatchers) often dug up recently buried corpses and extracted their teeth. Many of these came from the dead buried in hospital fields. The pulled teeth often carried contagious diseases such as TB or syphilis, and infected the new owners without their knowing.

Aboriginal Australians still have an interesting way of curing toothache. They heat up a bit of barbed wire and thrust it into the decayed tooth, killing the nerve immediately.

BELOW **These dentures for the lower jaw consist of human teeth set into hippopotamus ivory. It is possible that the teeth are "Waterloo Teeth," from that famous battlefield.**

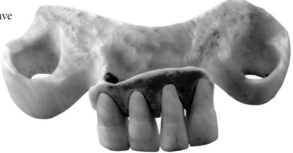

GOUT

One of the most revolting cures for a medical ailment ever written would have to be that given by Lorenz Fries to cure gout in 1518. His remedy involved roasting a fat old goose that was stuffed with chopped kittens, lard, wax, flour, and incense. The whole lot had to be consumed by the patient and the pan dripping was to be rubbed on the inflamed regions.

Given that gout is caused by a buildup of uric acid due to rich living, Fries's cure could only have exacerbated the symptoms. Anybody who has experienced gout knows the misery it causes. Uric acid builds up or crystallizes in a joint, and the first symptoms are an uncomfortable heat and stiffness. This may occur in any joint, such the ball of the thumb, the wrists, or, commonly, the ankle and big toe. The minor discomfort soon progresses to a blinding pain, and whenever the joint is moved or touched, agony spears through the entire limb. The mildest and most sweet-tempered person can be transformed into a raging ogre at the onset of an attack.

Gout in History

Gout has definitely changed the course of history. The Romans were notorious for their use of lead in their water systems and one of the side effects of lead poisoning was an inability to flush uric acid from the system due to inflammation of the kidney. Gout seems to have occurred in almost epidemic proportions among the Roman upper classes. Claudius, Nero, Caligula, and Tiberius are recorded as having gout-like symptoms and gout-inspired tantrums that led to many executions and poor decisions.

A much more solid case can be made for the fate of the Spanish Empire under Charles V (1500–58). Cursed with the Habsburg lip (a protruding lower jaw developed over centuries of inbreeding), he found it difficult to chew. Nevertheless, Charles loved his meat and drink, and ordered a huge drinking cup that required four handles. His gout was so bad that during the war with France in 1551, the emperor was unable to take to the field and lost a series of engagements that culminated in the loss of Metz. This could be argued to be a key event in the decline of the Spanish Holy Roman Empire, and Charles was forced to abdicate. In his retirement, the gout escalated; he had to be carried around in a sedan chair, and ramps were installed in his palaces. In 2006, one of Charles's fingers was examined by a Spanish medical team, and it was revealed that the acid was so pervasive that it had crystallized in his finger joints, destroying them and penetrating into his flesh.

RIGHT **An English treaty with Portugal had a nasty side effect for many English gentlemen. The ready access to port led to an epidemic of gout.**

Gout also had a role to play in Britain losing her American colonies. British statesman William Pitt the Elder (1708–88) was a firm advocate for preserving the union with the American territories. It was during his absences from parliament that the Stamp Act was

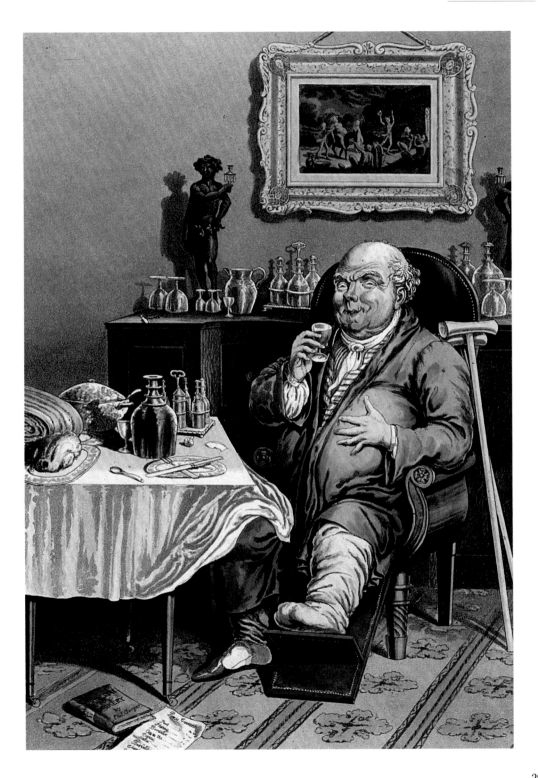

passed in 1765, with the intention of taxing the colonies. He returned from his attack of gout and had the law repealed. But during a subsequent onset of the debilitating condition and a repeat of his earlier absence, another levy was passed on colonial imports of tea, leading to the Boston Tea Party of 1773, which precipitated the American Revolution.

Common Cures for Gout

If gout is allowed to flourish unchecked, it can cause malformation and atrophy of digits. The first evidence of the condition is found in Egyptian mummies from approximately 4000 BCE. Otzi the Iceman discovered in the Italian Alps in 1990 is believed to have lived approximately 5,300 years ago. He had tattoos covering joints where gout often occurs, perhaps hinting at a ritual cure used many thousands of years in the past. Ancient Chinese treated gout with acupuncture and a form of cupping, where herbs were burnt in ceramic cones above the inflammation.

One of the first recorded references to gout is found in Homer's *Iliad*. Relating events of around 1200 BCE, he describes the experiences of the Trojan warrior Anchises whose toe was struck by lightning from Zeus, rendering him unable to walk. Hippocrates, the Greek physician, was the first to accurately describe the condition and wrote how long-term sufferers had atrophied joints caused by the long-term rheumatic effects of gout. He

BELOW If left untreated, gout can cause disfiguring tophi, painful lesions in the cartilage that eat away at the sufferer's bones.

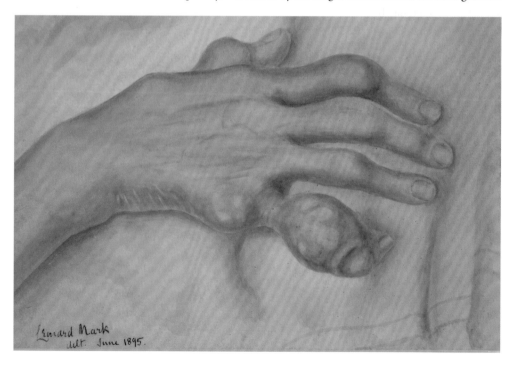

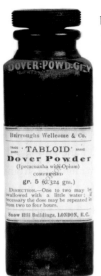

Burroughs Wellcome & Co.

'TABLOID' BRAND
Dover Powder
(Ipecacuanha with Opium)
COMPRESSED
gr. 5 (0.324 gm.)

DIRECTION.—One to two may be swallowed with a little water; if necessary the dose may be repeated in from two to four hours.

Snow Hill Buildings, LONDON, E.C.

believed the condition was caused by an imbalance of the four humors of the body and resulted in one of the humors accumulating, or "dropping" (*gutta* is Latin for "drop," leading to the name "gout") in the joints. This belief led medieval practitioners, who still followed this archaic medical orthodoxy, to prescribe bleeding and enemas. Another common cure was to "take the waters," and from 1597 an Act of Parliament made the waters of the thermal spa at Bath, England, available to all comers. These were fairly benign treatments. Other practitioners believed that ingesting boiled wolf was good for curing gout. Human fat blended with opium was thought to do the same.

In 1653 Nicholas Culpeper recommended a blend of horseradish and elder to be smeared on the affected area. In 1732 Thomas Dover invented his Dover Powder, which he claimed would banish all pain within two hours. Considering that this was basically powdered opium, it no doubt had this effect.

LEFT **Dover Powder could alleviate pain but led to addiction if overused, as it was an extremely strong opiate.**

In 1763 the first real breakthrough with the treatment of gout occurred when the Viennese physician Baron von Störck used an extract from the plant autumn crocus (*Colchicum autumnale*) to alleviate the symptoms. This was found to be an alkaloid that broke down the acid and it is still used in some modern-day treatments.

BELOW **Extract of autumn crocus is still used to cure gout: an example of a folk remedy that provided a real cure for a medical complaint.**

The stereotypical victim of gout, a stout and florid man given to overindulgence in rich meat and drink, was proved to be accurate in the 20th century. Research revealed that meat, seafood, and the darker-colored alcoholic drinks, such as claret and port, are most likely to trigger an attack. These drinks were most popular in the 1700s, which was no doubt gout's heyday.

Modern treatments act to either limit the amount of uric acid created or increase the amount that is excreted. By combining these treatments with a stiff course of anti-inflammatories, most modern attacks can be quickly bought under control.

Other cures for rheumatic conditions such as gout were to sleep next to a dog, which would then take on your condition, or else carry in your pocket a raw potato.

SCURVY

During the Age of Exploration (1500s to 1800s) as many as two million European sailors were struck down with scurvy.

The first sign a sailor experienced may have been the reopening of an old wound. The healed flesh would redden, become swollen, and then begin exuding blood and fluid. This was the first sign of a catastrophic breakdown of the body's systems. Scurvy occurs when a lack of ascorbic acid (vitamin C) effectively stops cell renewal, causing the sufferer's body to begin rotting. Other symptoms were swollen and spongy purplish gums, loose teeth, blood exuding from pores or hair follicles, bloody vomit, lassitude, putrescent sores, and finally heart failure and death. Gums often became so swollen that they covered the teeth in an oily, painful abscess, making it impossible for the victim to eat.

The worst aspect of this condition was perhaps the stench. As the sufferer's body rotted away, a reek of decaying, gangrenous flesh and fetid breath was exuded. Few things could be worse than sitting below decks in a cramped cabin becalmed in the tropics while your shipmates rotted around you in the tropical heat. One unnamed 16th-century sailor wrote:

It rotted all my gums, which gave out a black and putrid blood. My thighs and lower legs were black and gangrenous, and I was forced to use a knife each day to cut into the flesh in order to release this black and foul blood. I also used my knife on my gums, which were livid and growing over my teeth . . . When I had cut away the dead flesh and caused much black blood to flow, I rinsed my mouth and my teeth with my urine, rubbing them very hard . . . And the unfortunate thing was that I could not eat, desiring more to swallow than chew . . . Many of our people died from it every day, and we saw the bodies thrown into the sea constantly, three or four at a time. For the most part they died without aid given to them, expiring behind some case or chest, their eyes and the soles of their feet gnawed away by rats.

—UNNAMED 16TH-CENTURY SAILOR

LEFT **This man is prematurely aged by scurvy. The symptoms included waxen complexion, loose teeth, lack of energy, and skin sores.**

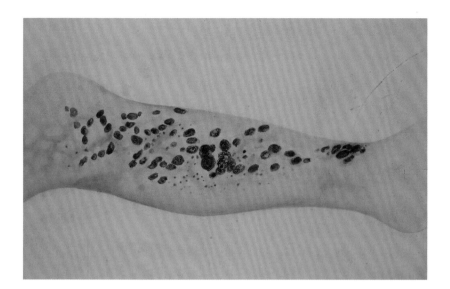

Surgeons at the time thought scurvy was an imbalance within the four humors. Black bile was seen as the culprit, as the symptoms always involved black blood, bile, vomit, and diarrhea. Other suggested causes were kissing women ashore, unwholesome miasmas, or just a mysterious infection.

ABOVE This patient's leg shows hemorrhaging below the skin, leading to bloody open sores. In extreme cases, internal organs might rupture.

Whole fleets could be devastated. In 1497, Vasco da Gama lost 100 members of the 160 crew who had set out to voyage around the Cape of Good Hope. In 1519 another great Portuguese explorer, Ferdinand Magellan, set out to circumnavigate the globe. Of the three ships and 250 men that sailed, only one ship and 18 men survived. Most died while becalmed in the Pacific and Indian Oceans, far removed from fresh food.

As European dominance of the oceans grew, so did their navies. Scurvy became a widespread scourge. During the Seven Years' War (1756–63), 184,899 British sailors were in service, 1,512 died in battle, and 133,708 died from disease, mainly scurvy.

The British naval rations at the time were admired by other states. Cheese, bacon, butter, biscuit, beer, and rum were provided in abundance, but of course fresh fruit and vegetables could not be preserved and were not always available.

Oranges and Lemons

It was the 1740 expedition by Sir George Anson to circumnavigate the globe that led to a cure for scurvy and, incidentally, the first clinical trial comparing control groups and monitoring inputs. Setting out with eight ships and 2,000 men, he returned in 1744 with only one ship and crew remaining. Scurvy had killed most of the deceased, and sometimes ten seamen would perish in one day.

Vitamin C is essential for the human body. It allows the synthesis of collagen, which is vital for creating new cells and generating connective tissues and bone mass. Lack of vitamin C leads to the steady erosion of muscle tissue and to weakening of the immune system.

Several remedies were available, and sailors knew that eating tropical fruit kept the illness at bay. Jacques Cartier (1491–1557), who claimed Canada for France, noticed that Indians who had scurvy would drink tea made of sprouting pine needles. After a week they would recover, and Cartier recommended this remedy. Other herbal remedies abounded but none were officially recognized by any admiralty.

This all changed after the Scot James Lind (1716–94) wrote his *Treatise of the Scurvy* in 1753. During May 1747 Lind, a naval physician, had 12 of his sick shipmates confined to the forepeak, where he conducted the first clinical trial in history. All were given the basic diet of gruel, mutton broth, pudding, and sago with currants. Beyond this he varied their diet with recommended cures for scurvy. Two received a quart of cider, two had oil of vitriol, two had vinegar, two had seawater, and two had a blend of herbs including myrrh and garlic, while the last received oranges and lemons. The pair on oranges and lemons were cured within the week while the others

BELOW James Lind conducted the first modern clinical trials to determine the best cure for scurvy and saved countless lives.

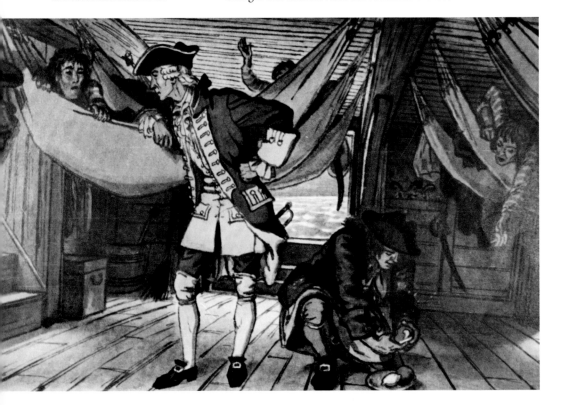

How to Cure a Hernia

Guy de Chauliac (ca. 1300–60) wrote the influential work *Chirurgia Magna*. Concentrating on anatomy, he sought to cure the world's ills. A hernia occurs when an organ pushes through an opening in the muscle or tissue that holds it in. De Chauliac suggested as a cure that the first responsibility of the doctor was to give laxatives, emetics, and suppositories to produce regular bowel movements. Regular bleeding was to be administered. The patient was to avoid fruit, wholegrain bread, fish, cheese, port, beans, and radishes. Wine and water were expressly forbidden. The patient was then to be hung by his feet to reduce the hernia. After hanging upside down for several hours, he was to be strapped in plaster and confined to bed for 50 days.

By 1776 the treatment of hernias had not improved. For the naturalist Gilbert White of Selborne, England, the recommended cure was to find a pollarded ash sapling and split it down the middle. It was then held open with the use of wedges and the patient was passed between the split sections. The surgeon then had to bandage the tree with a stiff plaster. If the tree healed, so would the patient. On the Continent hernias had, up until the 16th century, rather unpleasant implications for male sufferers: surgeons believed that if it was necessary to operate on a male patient, he had to be castrated first!

continued to suffer. The Admiralty was convinced and several years later an ounce of lemon juice mixed with sugar was issued to all hands after six weeks at sea.

Lind's recommendations weren't the only scurvy preventative. When Captain Cook's *Endeavour* sailed from England in 1768, it had 98 men on board. The ship returned in 1771 minus 38 crew, who had died of various illnesses and misfortunes, but none had died of scurvy. Cook made sure to supply his crew with as much fresh food as possible and at Rio de Janeiro, Brazil, each crewman received 20 pounds (9 kg) of raw onions! When fresh food was not available he supplied sauerkraut (pickled cabbage). At first the crew were wary, but when they saw the officers tucking in they decided it couldn't be all bad, and soon the cabbage had to be rationed.

THE BLACK DEATH

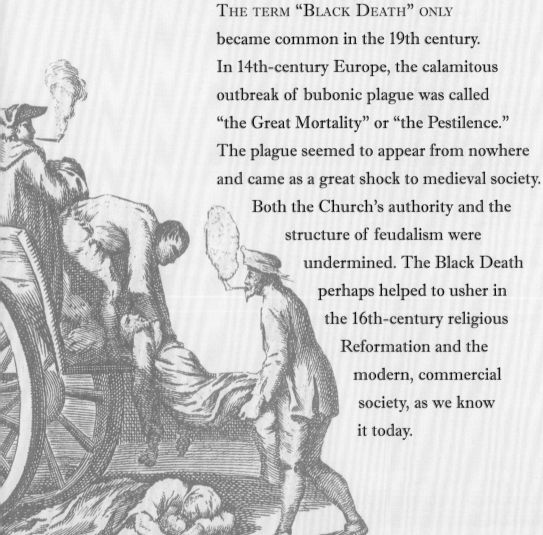

THE TERM "BLACK DEATH" ONLY became common in the 19th century. In 14th-century Europe, the calamitous outbreak of bubonic plague was called "the Great Mortality" or "the Pestilence." The plague seemed to appear from nowhere and came as a great shock to medieval society. Both the Church's authority and the structure of feudalism were undermined. The Black Death perhaps helped to usher in the 16th-century religious Reformation and the modern, commercial society, as we know it today.

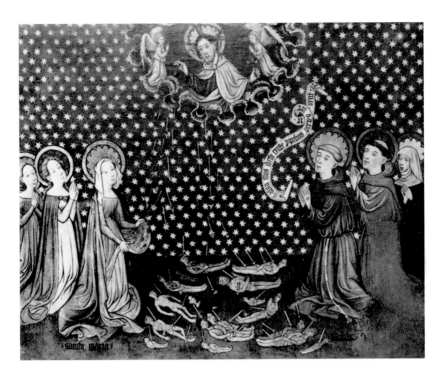

GOD'S WRATH

The shell-shocked population of medieval Europe, as well as the earlier Byzantines, believed that the plague was evidence of God's wrath for their fornication, blasphemy, greed, heresy, and all the other activities that the Catholic Church deemed to be sinful. Such was the horror of the disease that it could not be attributed to a kind, benevolent God but one spewing forth bile, hate, and everlasting damnation.

Those who believe in the concept of "intelligent design" (a philosophical view that assumes the universe is shaped by an intelligent being rather than natural selection) would have to agree that the plague bacterium, *Yersinia pestis*, is a marvelous biological killing machine able to infect and overwhelm both the respiratory system and the cardiovascular system. The rod-shaped bacterium is named after the Swiss scientist Alexandre Yersin, who discovered it in 1894. This lethal bacterium can infect the body in three main ways: Bubonic plague infects the lymphatic symptom, pneumonic plague attacks the airways, while septicemic plague occurs when the bacteria invade the bloodstream.

BUBONIC PLAGUE

The bubonic form of the plague was perhaps the most common infection in medieval times, but only exists in rare pockets today. In the initial outbreak probably 70 percent of people who contracted the disease died within four to seven days, although in later outbreaks this death toll would have been reduced as immunity within a population increased.

The disease caused agonizing symptoms affecting the entire body. The infection would spread throughout the host's lymph glands. The first signs of infections were "tokens"—small lumps found near the lymph glands. The neck, underarms, and groin were the most common sites. These tokens were merely the harbingers of the buboes that developed from them, which caused agonizing pain with even the slightest movement. These lumps ranged from the size of an almond to the size of an orange, and were filled with a vile concoction of clotted blood, pus, and suppurating flesh. Accompanying the tokens were mild fevers that would become raging attacks of delirium as temperatures could soar to 102° Fahrenheit (39° Celsius). The disease often attacked the nervous system, leading to compulsive jerking, laughing, screaming, and a whole host of other distressing symptoms, such as muscle cramps, seizures, vomiting, fainting, extreme lethargy, coughing, and swollen joints. The other common sign of plague was the large blue or black blotches that appeared just under the skin, indicating hemorrhages and corrupted flesh. Necrosis would also occur, which is when muscle mass and organs begin to die, allowing dead cells to overwhelm the immune system and leading to multiple organ failure. Gangrene could set in on the rotting flesh, and delirium followed by coma were often the last symptoms before death.

RIGHT **Physicians believed that the plague was airborne. They used masks stuffed with sweet-smelling herbs to ward off the disease.**

BELOW **Small tokens in the armpits, groin, and neck are the first signs of bubonic plague. These expand into buboes as the lymphatic system becomes host to the plague bacilli.**

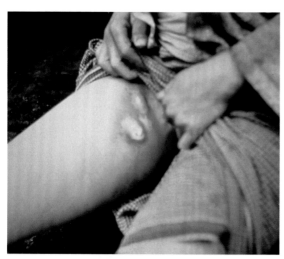

If the buboes burst of their own accord within seven days, patients had some chance of surviving—if secondary infections didn't finish them off.

The 14th-century writer Giovanni Boccaccio, from Florence, Italy, described the plague as follows:

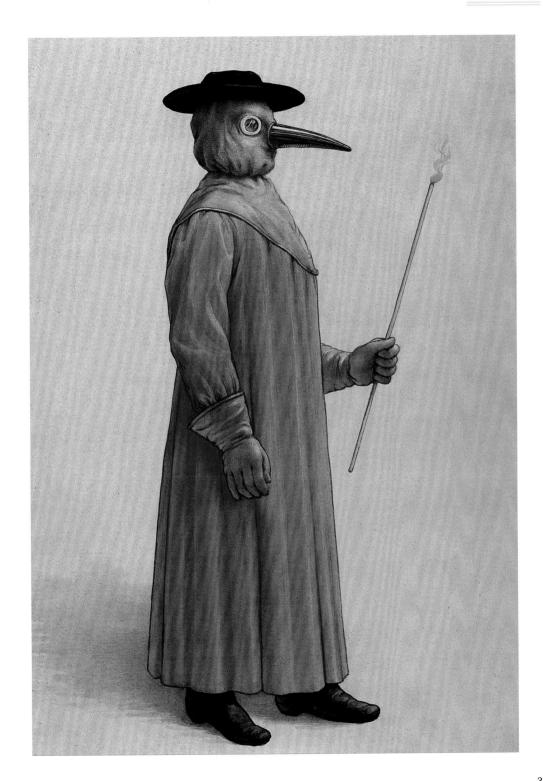

The disease began both in men and women with certain small swellings around the groin or armpit. These then grew to the size of a small orange or an egg, thereabouts, and were commonly called tumors. These tumors rapidly spread from the two parts named to cover the body. Soon after this the symptoms altered and black or purple spots emerged on the arms or thighs or any other part of the body, some times a few large ones, and other times many little ones. These spots were seen as a sure sign of death, just as the original tumor had been and still was. The sick gave the disease to those who were uninfected whenever they became close; the disease was as violent as a fire catching upon an oily rag. It was even worse. Even the act of speaking to those who were infected or to touch the clothes or anything else that the sick had touched or worn spread the disease.

—*Decameron*, Giovanni Boccaccio, trans. Jonathan J. Moore

Pneumonic Plague

The bubonic plague, which struck the lymphatic system, was far eclipsed in horrific lethality by the pneumonic plague, where the bacteria infected the respiratory system and could be transmitted by coughing. Before the Black Death, the European medical establishment blamed pestilential air for many infections. While this was largely based on a poorly understood idea of transmission of diseases, for the pneumonic plague they were tragically accurate. In some cases the bacilli infected the lungs, leading to infected airways and allowing the plague to be spread in minute droplets of sputum, whenever the patient coughed or sneezed. This dreadful variant could kill in less than 36 hours and produced a fatality rate of about 99 percent.

BELOW *Yersinia pestis*, **the bacterium that causes the bubonic plague, is one of the deadliest organisms on earth. Over millions of years it has evolved to live in a variety of hosts.**

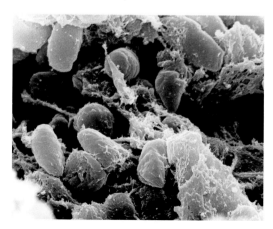

The initial symptom is coughing, which degenerates into coughing blood. This is followed by fever, headache, shortness of breath, chest pains, and watery sputum. The entire respiratory system shuts down as it is overwhelmed with fluids that cannot be expelled from the lungs, and heart failure often follows. This form of the plague is echoed in the common nursery rhyme "Ring Around the Rosie." The line a "pocket full of posies" represents the bunches of aromatics

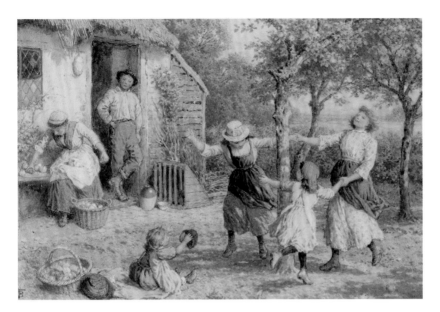

that people would hold under their noses to try and avoid sickness (the price of lavender escalated during outbreaks). "A-tishoo, a-tishoo" represents the coughing and sneezing, and "we all fall down" is self-explanatory.

ABOVE **"Ring Around the Rosie," now a harmless childhood rhyme, describes the lethal pneumonic plague that killed 99 percent of those infected.**

Chroniclers of the epidemic mention that to be coughed upon or to share the air of the sick often led to rapid onset of death. It appears that many of the largest towns in Europe were infected with both bubonic and pneumonic plague as it ravaged the population during the outbreak from 1347 to 1352.

SEPTICEMIC PLAGUE

One of the plague stories often told during medieval times is of people who are fine when they get up but are dead by lunchtime. These may be referring to the third and deadliest version of the disease: septicemic plague. This too is insect-borne, but rather than attacking the lymph nodes it attacks and overwhelms the bloodstream, which within two hours is swarming with the plague bacilli. This leads to multiple tiny blood clots that cause cells and portions of the body to die due to lack of oxygen. Since the clotting agents are overwhelmed, blood begins seeping into muscle tissue and organs, leading to red or black blotches on the skin and eventual organ failure. Other symptoms include abdominal pain, bleeding from the mouth, nose, or rectum, diarrhea, nausea, shock, difficulty in breathing, and gangrene, as the extremities die

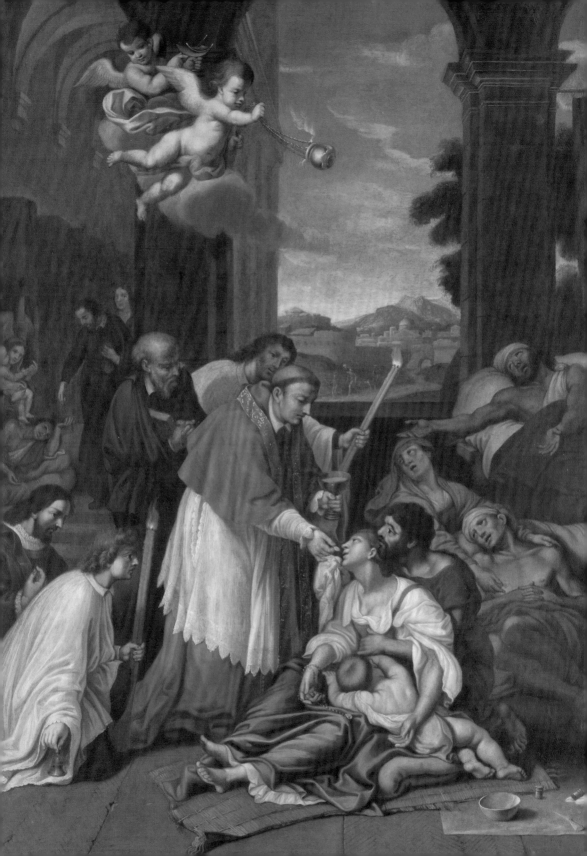

due to lack of oxygen, particularly the fingers, toes, and nose. The sufferer expires within 24 hours, sometimes within as little as 4 hours, before buboes can arise and/or the lungs can be infected. Bacteria-rich blood is, of course, perfect for transmission of the plague when the flea makes a meal of it before moving on to new hosts.

A Ratty Problem

The bacteria begin as harmless passengers in the guts of small mammals such as rats and mice, before spreading into the bloodstream. Here they will kill the host but ensure that they survive in other parasites.

Fleas suck in the infected rodent blood and then the diabolical genius of the bacteria reveals itself. The fleas fill themselves with the infected blood but, rather than passing through to the gut of the flea to be digested, the bacteria cause the blood to clot, making the poor flea ravenously hungry and thirsty. The flea becomes a frenzied insect feeding machine. In its crazed need for sustenance, the flea jumps onto another host and bites into its skin to try and draw in more blood. Before it does so, it injects from its throat some of the previous host's undigested blood complete with the bacterium *Yersinia pestis*, so infecting the new host.

The cunning strategies of this ruthless killer aren't finished. Just as the poor flea is about to expire from lack of nutrition, the bacterium allows the stomach to empty itself into the guts of its host, enabling the insect to replenish its energy stores. After a period of time it gets up to its old tricks and clots again, sending the poor flea off on another murderous rampage.

During medieval times the flea came into contact with the black rat (*Rattus rattus*), and this is when *Yersinia pestis* became a danger to human populations. Familiar with human habitats, black rats were particularly at home living in ships. Originally a tree-dwelling rat, the rodents are able to climb ropes and rigging with ease ensuring that they could easily disperse from infected ships and spread the plague. Many people who lived through the plague suspected the disease was spread through cloth being traded on boats, or else was contagious from the clothes of the infected; in a sense they were right. In a dense, close-knit population with only rudimentary hygiene, one flea could be the epicenter of a vast infectious outbreak.

LEFT This picture represents St. Charles Borromeo tending to a plague victim. In reality many powerful churchmen fled into the countryside, abandoning their flock.

BELOW The sight of black rats expiring out in the open was one of the first signs that the plague was approaching. The bacteria only kept rats alive long enough to spread to new victims.

FILTHY TIMES

MEDIEVAL HYGIENE standards left a lot to be desired. Towns did not have sewerage systems and neither were they equipped with fresh water supplies.

The British slang term for toilet, "the loo," comes from the French phrase *guardez l'eau*, which translates as "watch out for the water," the phrase commonly heard as chamber pots were emptied out into the street. Some homes had indoor privies built into their outer walls, but these were little more than a hole cut in the floor, which dropped the waste into the alley below. The effluent could either stay and rot where it fell, or be washed into local streams and waterways. The amount of waste was staggering. In medieval London alone it is estimated that 55 tons (50 metric tonnes) of human excrement had to be removed daily, and this does not even factor in the waste from cats, dogs, and horses.

The Church condemned bathing as immoral, and medieval doctors taught that diseases were carried through the water and passed on through the pores of the skin. Many medieval Europeans forewent bathing altogether. As a rule, the wealthier you were, the more

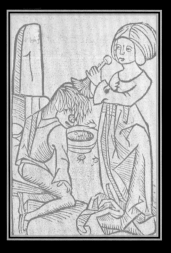

you tended to bathe. Medieval nobility bathed regularly, about twice a year on average. Some risk-takers even bathed once a month. A more cautious type, Queen Isabella I of Spain (1451–1504), claimed to have bathed only twice in her lifetime—when she was born, and on her wedding day. The story of Thomas Becket, Archbishop of Canterbury from 1162 to 1170, tells an even fouler tale. When his murdered corpse was undressed, an eyewitness was shocked to see a mass of vermin that "boiled over like water in a simmering cauldron."

To compensate for the stench, Europe's nobles would coat themselves in perfume and satchels of flowers. The effect was less than glamorous. Ironically, it was the fear of disease that kept Europeans from bathing, but it was their lack of hygiene that attracted rats infested with fleas, literally exploding with the bacterium *Yersinia pestis*, which had made its way to Europe via East Asia in the 1340s. This was the cause of the bubonic plague.

ABOVE Hygiene was not always a priority in medieval society. Disease was thought to spread through noxious vapors called "miasma," infecting the clean and dirty alike.

THE SPREAD OF THE PLAGUE

Hunter–gatherer communities before the Neolithic period (New Stone Age) in approximately 10,000 BCE may have first caught the plague from small rodents. A sick animal is slower than its healthy counterparts and easier to catch. Opportunistic hunting may have led to cross-species transfer of the disease and some nomadic bands may have been infected. However, it was only when humanity became highly urbanized that the plague emerged as one of the most lethal crowd diseases (see Introduction) ever.

The bubonic plague is suspected to have arisen in the ancient world. There is a possibility that this disease attacked the Philistines at Ashod in the 11th century BCE and that there was a terrible outbreak of the plague in Hellenistic Egypt and North Africa in 200 BCE.

These events paled into insignificance before the dreadful effect that an outbreak had on the Eastern (Byzantine) and Western Roman Empires in the 6th century CE. So devastating was this outbreak that it put the final nail in the coffin of the Western Roman Empire, while depopulating so much of Europe that it was

BELOW **The Philistines settled in the Levant in the late Bronze Age. They dominated their neighbors with sophisticated weapons but these did not protect them from the plague.**

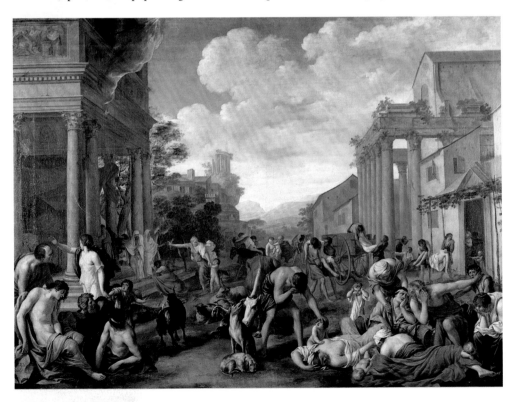

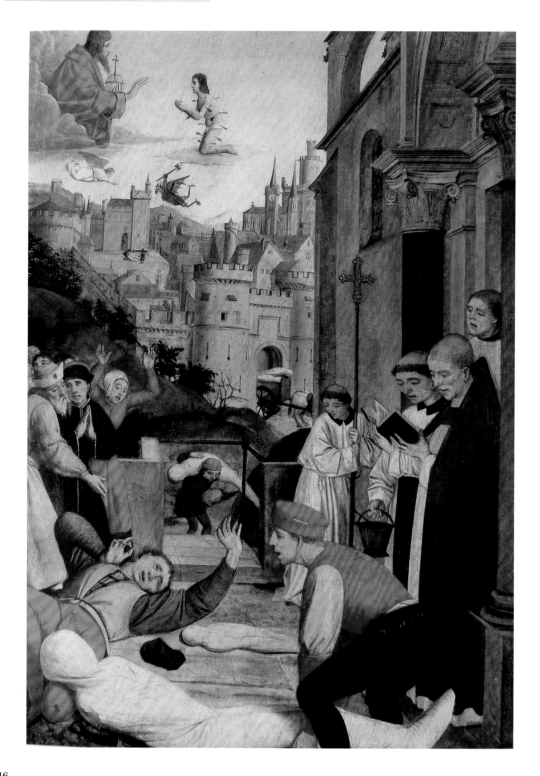

partly blamed for the onset of the Dark Ages. This outbreak was known in Constantinople in the time of Emperor Justinian (483–565) as the "Great Dying."

Emerging from the trade routes leading out of Egypt, the "pestilence by which the whole human race came near to be annihilated" reached Constantinople in 542 CE. The reported symptoms leave no room for doubt that this was an outbreak of the bubonic plague. It began with a fever before swollen lymph glands led to buboes in the armpits, groin, and neck. Lethargy and hallucinations were then observed before most victims died within five days. The bubonic plague then morphed into the pneumonic plague and people died within one or two days spitting blood and coughing out their lungs.

Just as in the later medieval plague, the structure of society seemed to come unglued. Crime was unchecked and there were so many bodies that they were impossible to dispose of. The roofs of the great defensive towers on the walls of Constantinople were removed and the bodies were stacked in them. Others were thrown on rafts and rowed out to sea or burned on funeral pyres that blackened the sky.

Over 40 percent of Constantinople's population died and the plague swept around the Mediterranean coast before heading inland into Europe, where similar depredations occurred. North Africa and the Middle East were decimated and the plague reached China in 610 CE.

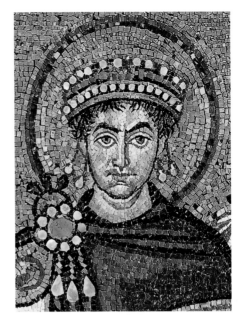

ABOVE Justinian sought to reconquer the Western Roman Empire from the barbarians. But even his famous general Belisarius could not hold back the plague.

LEFT European cities struggled to dispose of the mountains of corpses created by the Black Death. Hasty burials in simple winding sheets became a common sight.

The Eastern Roman Emperor Justinian's efforts to reclaim the Western Roman Empire from 543 to 540 CE were largely futile and the weakened states around the Mediterranean became tempting targets for Islamic conquest. Europe, which had experienced warfare for at least a hundred years as the Western Empire collapsed under the weight of barbarian invasions, was further depopulated by this outbreak, leading to an unprecedented flight to the countryside. Large-scale urban settlements such as Rome were reduced to pitiful remnants of their former glory and the population dispersed into smaller rural settlements, living under the authority of tribal leaders. It wasn't until 700 years later that Europe's population had recovered to such an extent that it became once again a fertile target for the bubonic plague.

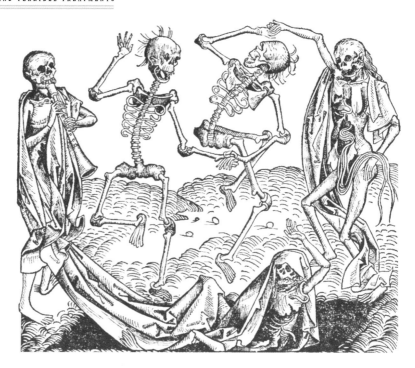

ABOVE *The Dance of Death* (1493) by **Michael Wolgemut. This allegorical engraving depicting the universality of death seems particularly relevant to the plague: no matter their status in life, all were susceptible to the deadly disease.**

The Plague in Asia

The plague was heralded by drought, earthquakes, flood, and famine in northern China before 1320. Many rural populations were affected by dreadful droughts along the Hoai River, followed by locust plagues descending from the grasslands to the north. A massive flood killed at least 400,000 people while an earthquake, "subterraneous thunder," in Canton killed at least another 5 million. These disasters were merely a prelude to a greater catastrophe that would ravage China's populations for the next two decades.

Endemic to small rodents in the south of China near the border with Indochina, the plague bacteria somehow leaped the species divide between rodent and human. The first known outbreak was reported by 1318 in Pagan, a town located within modern-day Myanmar (Burma) near the border with India. For some reason the dreadful disease moved north and by 1320 massive outbreaks were reported in Yunnan and Xian. The region around Wuchang was devastated in 1332, and throughout the next two decades the plague reappeared throughout eastern and northern China, reaching as far as Beijing.

The Yuan dynasty was fatally weakened by the continual outbreaks and most Chinese thought it was clear evidence that this Mongol dynasty had lost the "Mandate of Heaven." Sadly for Europe, the Yuan rulers were only an outpost of the mighty Mongol Empire founded by Genghis Khan and trade routes curling throughout this

Population Decimated

Ice cores measuring human carbon emissions from the last millennium reveal two large dips in the amount of fuel being burned by human activity. These indicate two drastic reductions in the human population. One was in the first half of the 16th century when smallpox, measles, steel, and gunpowder caused a catastrophic collapse in the indigenous population of the Americas. The previous, more drastic, drop was when the bubonic plague ravaged populations throughout temperate Asia and Europe from 1320 to 1353.

empire, such as the Silk Road, brought the storm of pestilence into the heart of Europe. No doubt fleas traveling on expensive silks and woolen garments along these once prosperous trade routes carried the disease. By 1346 the Mongol warriors of the Khanate of The Golden Horde were being infected by the pestilence.

The main field army of this khanate was prosecuting a siege against the Genoese trading outpost of Caffa (Kaffa) situated on the eastern side of the Crimea in the Black Sea. The plague ravaged this peninsula and at least 85,000 are estimated to have died within the area in 1346 alone. The Mongol soldiers also began to succumb and it was decided to call off the siege. Before they did this, they catapulted infected corpses into the fortified settlement, feeling that the Christians should not escape the divine and deadly visitation.

The Plague Reaches Europe

The Italians in Caffa took desperate measures: They hauled the festering dead to the town's quay and threw them into the ocean as quickly as possible. But not quickly enough! Soon the plague broke out within Caffa. Realizing the game was up, the Genoese survivors loaded all their trade goods into some galleys and rowed very fast toward the Mediterranean. They infected Constantinople and Sicily in 1347, and had hit the European mainland by 1348. People in Messina were horrified to see a galley arriving in their port with only a few sick and diseased seamen staggering ashore to die, followed by a horde of rats. Another report from a Flemish chronicler reported three galleys putting in at Genoa laden with spices, riches, and sick sailors. Almost immediately infections broke out in the Genoese population, so the galleys were driven away with burning arrows and catapults, driving them to seek aid in other ports, thereby spreading the disease even more rapidly.

While these stories are probably apocryphal, it is nevertheless obvious that goods brought from the Black Sea were responsible for the plague's transmission to Europe. By the end of 1347, the plague had engulfed Corsica and Sardinia and reached Marseille in France. By mid-1348 most of France and Spain was infected and by December 1349 England and the German states had experienced the full horror of the deadly disease. In England, the course of the disease moved in a simple northwest axis, while Germany was threatened by the disease crossing the Rhineland, as well as moving from the east through the Balkans and the Hungarian plateau. Egypt was struck in 1347 and by 1351 the disease had reached Aden at the bottom of the Arabian Peninsula. These populations were ravaged, with half to two-thirds of the people perishing as the deadly scythe decimated the population.

Europe lost at least half of its population, and North Africa and the Islamic states of the East lost one-third to half of their people, as did India. The original source of the Black Death in the 14th century—China—saw its population drop from 120 million to approximately 65 million. The remnant Byzantine Empire was decimated, allowing its gradual overthrow by both Christian and Muslim enemies. Constantinople fell to the Ottomans in 1453.

BELOW **The plague of Florence in 1348. Churches were forbidden from ringing their bells during funerals as it demoralized the population.**

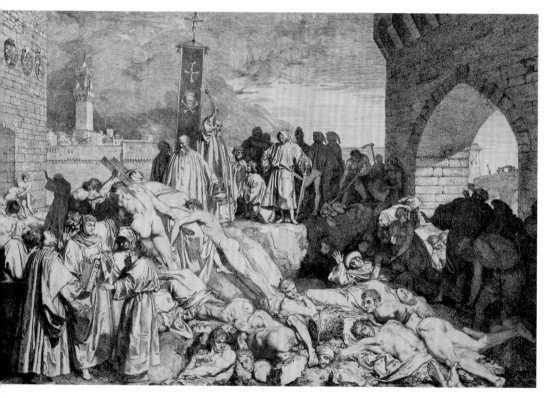

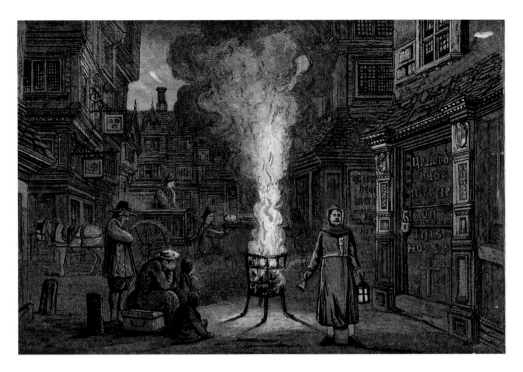

BUBOES, CARBUNCLES, AND PUS

Writing in *Loimographia: An Account of the Great Plague of London in the Year 1665*, Dr. William Boghurst provided a vivid description of the unpleasant symptoms of the plague, with several chapters devoted to his incredibly detailed knowledge of buboes and carbuncles.

Today, we define a carbuncle as a large abscess or infection that has several openings where pus and blood ooze out of the skin. Or else it can be a cluster of suppurating abscesses and boils. Boghurst has a differing definition and believes they are named carbuncles because they look like large, raised black or blue boils that may be caused by burning with a hot iron that has been heated with "carbon," or coal. His description of them is vivid. They break out anywhere on the fleshy parts of the body, but never the head or stomach, and are blue or black. They begin as a fiery red swelling that rises to become a large black protuberance, sometimes with one or many pus-filled white dots on top. These black growths then became stiff and hard, and excruciating to touch. Elsewhere he noted that some carbuncles were large swellings "the size of a head" covering large areas of the skin, with a fiery red circle around them raised one inch (2.5 cm) from the surrounding skin or recessed ⅜ inch (1 cm) below. Sometimes the entire surface began to rot off,

ABOVE The Great Plague of London, 1665, saw municipal authorities locking up entire households even if only one person was infected. "Watchers" were employed to ensure no one escaped.

leaving large pieces of flesh denuded of skin; and he noticed that if the core expelled its poison, the carbuncle would dry out harmlessly, leaving a tiny scar when it was completely healed. He noted that a patient who was constipated or had a fever with the carbuncles would most likely die, but the more fortunate survivors might have them exuding pus and fluids for six or seven weeks before they dried out. Sometimes the carbuncles would be hard and black on the surface, but rotting beneath and exuding a foul odor, leading to a slow death of several weeks.

The buboes' chief distinction from carbuncles according to the good Dr. Boghurst was that they would rise, not on the fleshy parts but in the groin, under the neck, and under the armpits. He also observed that sometimes they arose on the shoulder or breast, and these buboes would never burst but would rather disappear deeper into the flesh. The buboes that arose in the groin tended to be wedge-shaped with a high red ridge on the crest. If they came immediately to the surface as soon as the illness struck, they were favorably inclined to burst and heal, whereas the buboes that arose several days into the sickness would become more painful as the bacteria progressed and lingered. Some survivors suffered these buboes in their groin for up to three months before they finally worked their way to the surface. He describes how buboes around the neck and arms were less troublesome, and sometimes burst after two weeks, running for only two more days before they healed themselves. They rarely

BELOW The plague hit Napoleon's French army when he invaded Egypt in 1799. He proved his devotion to his men when he visited the plague hospital in Jaffa.

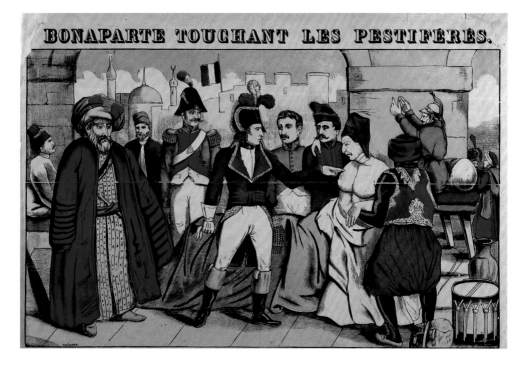

BONAPARTE TOUCHANT LES PESTIFÉRÉS.

leaked pus, more likely oozing a thin, bloody substance. If a patient appeared to be on the mend and the bubo in this area seemed to be getting better, a wise surgeon could give it a good squeeze and extract "a rope of thick, long, putrefied matter." These buboes were usually the size of a fist, and the old and "dry" flesh of the elderly would only have one or two, but those with "warm soft" flesh, such as children, could have four to six. Those who had tokens and buboes were most likely to die, while people who displayed late-coming growths or "white" buboes were likely to survive.

Finally, the good doctor described "blaines" or blisters. These were a little like carbuncles but quite small, with only a small, pus-filled core. They were usually quite benign, accompanied by a slight fever, and were only fatal if they were present with tokens. Obviously people who displayed these symptoms were blessed with a degree of immunity.

CURES AND PREVENTATIVES

Plague Doctors

"Where there's shit there's gold" runs an old saying. The same applies to the plague, where many medieval doctors tried to make their fortune by selling pamphlets and cures to a desperate public. While many priests and bishops fled to the countryside, doctors at least attempted to alleviate the sufferings of the locals. They often acted as advisors to town councils and their recommendations, such as keeping streets clean and storing foodstuffs hygienically, became routine in cities from London to Genoa. Hospitals became places of research and learning rather than repositories for the dying.

During the medieval period, the most commonly ascribed causes of the plague were miasmas and pestilential airs. These were thought to come from the sea, from swamps, from the dead, or to be sent by an angry God. Many preventatives suggested avoiding places where pestilential air could accumulate, and there were many recommendations to burn herbs and aromatics to disperse the noxious gasses. Smoking tobacco was touted as a possible cure and was considered particularly effective for young children. Cat and dog fur was seen as a likely emitter of vapors, and many municipalities organized mass killings of these animals as soon as plague tokens appeared in their community. This was, of course, a fatal error. Before poisons became readily available, the main means of keeping down rat numbers was predation by domestic or semi-domestic animals such as cats and dogs. Without them, rats were able to breed unchecked, spreading the deadly germs.

Given that the idea of bacteria and viruses had hardly occurred to medieval people, it is not surprising that they had no clue of how to cure or prevent the plague.

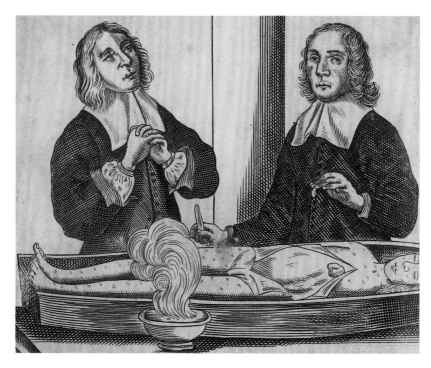

ABOVE **Doctors sought to understand what caused the plague. Without an understanding of germ theory, dissections such as this from 1666 could only reveal the symptoms.**

Many far-fetched and imaginative cures were designed. These fabulous concoctions had several things in common: They could only have worked as a placebo, and they required huge amounts of dead animals and plants cooked up in horrible concoctions.

In his *Loimographia*, Dr. Boghurst listed all the things that should be avoided if his patients wished to escape the plague. Poor hygiene isn't mentioned but he does blame the disease on lust, pride, whoring, profanity, profit, pleasure, usury, feasting, the theater, hypocrisy, greed, lack of charity, heresy, wine, beer, brandy, strong waters, amulets, charms, witchcraft, bathing, bleeding, purging, vomiting, swimming in rivers or ponds, and finally, getting emotional.

Boghurst does give good advice on what uninfected people should avoid if they want to stay healthy once the plague has taken hold. People should avoid killing cats or dogs (not because they kill rats but because they would be left where they fell, leading to further filth and odor), joining crowds, "especially" using linen from the deceased, lying near full graveyards, excrement of the dead, bad odors, and cobwebs.

Even during the 1665 plague, Peter Lillicrap understood market forces and printed a handbook called *A Collection of Seven and Fifty Approved Receipts* [recipes] *Good Against the Plague: Taken Out of the Five Books of that Renowned Dr. Don Alexes Secrets, for the Benefit of the Poorer Sort of People of These Nations.* Aimed at the lower end of the market, it was probably a real recipe for success from a commercial viewpoint, but maybe less so from a medical standpoint. Two of his medicines are quite harmless:

Take an onion and cut it into four pieces. Cut a piece out of each quarter and fill it with treacle. Wrap the rejoined onion in white linen and roast it in some coals. Once it is cooked squeeze out the juices and give the patient a spoonful and soon he would feel a whole lot better.

Grind some dried seeds from a bay tree and mix it with a little salt. As soon as the patient feels a fever he should mix this with some water and vinegar and have a good lie down covered with sheep skins. If symptoms persist, use wine instead of vinegar.

Later on Dr. Alexes gets a bit more imaginative:

Fill a glass one third full of treacle, one third full of spring water and one third full of the urine of a young boy virgin who exhibits good health. Drink this three days in a row. The Venetians swore by this cure.

The patient should drink good quality treacle and eat chestnuts. Then rub treacle on the buboes, cut a pigeon in half and lie the pigeon halves with the feather outwards on the growths. Once the pigeon flesh turns green it should be removed and squeezed. Any green juices that emerge from the pigeon have been sucked from the bubo.

Take the oldest oil you can get and boil it for several hours. Once this has been done put 50 scorpions per pound of oil into the mixture and cook it until it has reduced by a third. Once this has been done pull out the scorpions and strain the mixture through some cloth into another container and leave this in the sun for three months or in the ashes of a fire for four days. Once this has been done put in two ounces of Unicorn horn, one ounce of treacle and some pure water. Once a patient starts to feel bad, apply this lotion to the chest above the heart, the neck and the wrists there will be a "marvelous effect."
—A COLLECTION OF SEVEN AND FIFTY APPROVED RECEIPTS GOOD AGAINST THE PLAGUE, W. J., GENT.

No doubt this recipe explains why unicorns and scorpions are now very hard to find in the British Isles.

One other surefire cure was to pluck the feathers from the bottom of a chicken where "the egge doth emerge" and hold the beast against the buboes so that it can absorb all of the pestilence within.

THE SICKNESS IN THE FORM OF EVIL VAPORS ENTERED THROUGH THE PORES OF THE SKIN AND WAS CARRIED BY THE BLOOD TO THE HEART, BRAIN, AND LIVER. ONCE AT THE HEART, THE EVIL VAPORS WOULD BE EXPELLED TO THE HEART'S EMUNCTORIES, WHICH WERE LOCATED IN THE ARMPIT. IF THE PATIENT WAS NOT BLED THERE AT THE RIGHT TIME, THE POISON RACED TO THE LIVER...

RIGHT A 13th-century parchment purporting to explain the vascular system. It was believed that the lungs were responsible for the circulation of blood.

BELOW This illustration from 1675 shows a patient bleeding himself in order to lessen his symptoms. Such treatments were likely to be counterproductive.

Many medieval doctors recommended dead animals or different foodstuffs to be applied as a poultice to the affected areas to draw out the poison. Dried toads were a commonly ascribed remedy. Bloodletting was another common cure, but at that time it was a bit of a generic solution to a range of ills. Some doctors believed that they could lance parts of the body and actually intercept the noxious blood before it infected the whole body. A certain John of Burgundy evolved an entire science around the use of bleeding in 1365. Using some data known only to himself, John determined that dispersed around the body were "emunctories" which if bled at the correct time could expel poison. The sickness in the form of evil vapors entered through the pores of the skin and was carried by the blood to the heart, brain, and liver. Once at the heart, the evil vapors would be expelled to the heart's emunctories, which were located in the armpit. If the patient was not bled there at the right time, the poison raced to the liver before going to the liver's emunctory, which was of course the groin. From there it traveled to the brain and the ears. Certain veins in these areas needed to be lanced to expel the poison before too much damage was caused. No doubt some doctors following these guidelines advised that it was better to be safe than sorry and lance all of the possible veins.

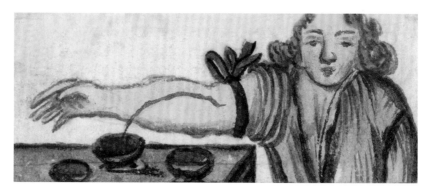

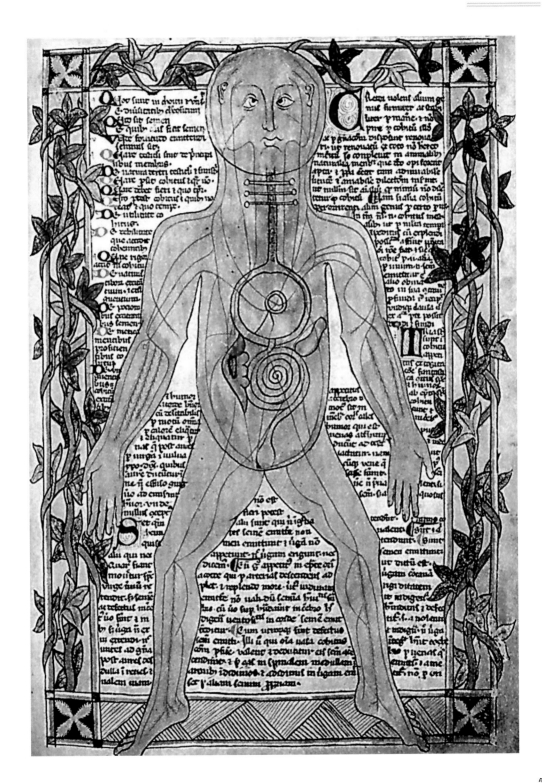

DISPOSAL OF THE DEAD

The sheer volume of putrescent corpses, many covered with burst, pus-filled buboes, blood, scabs, urine, and feces, overwhelmed the cemeteries and churches of the towns when the plague first struck Europe in the 14th century. Adding to the problem was the reluctance of any but the most desperate to handle the corpses for a fee, and the desire of most clergy members to flee from the plague spots into the countryside.

There is evidence that when the plague struck Eastern Europe, communities used older superstitions to try and stop its spread. Throughout this region mothers and their children who had died of the plague would be buried at crossroads. Mothers would be laid to rest with their children enfolded in their crossed arms, in emulation of the Virgin Mary and Child.

In Venice, Italy, it was estimated that 600 victims were dying each day at the height of the plague in 1348. A panel was empowered to deal with the mountains of dead in such a way as would not infect the waterways. Certain islands, including what is now called the Lido, were selected to bury the dead, and it was stipulated that the corpses had to be buried under at least 5 feet (150 cm) of earth. Special plague barges were established to transport the dead. Beggars were forbidden from carrying out their usual practice of displaying dead bodies in the streets in order to solicit alms, so that passersby would take pity on them. In Siena, the municipal authorities didn't have as much power as the Venetians and no workers could be found to bury

BELOW Only the poorest of the poor could be enticed to bury the dead. Many corpses were left to rot, particularly in the countryside.

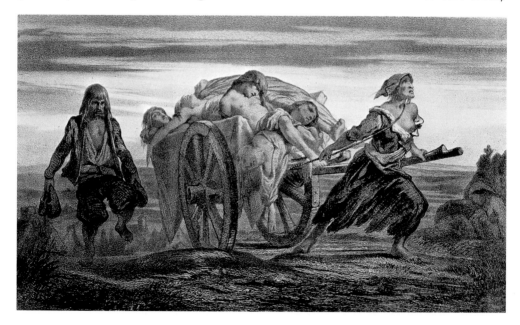

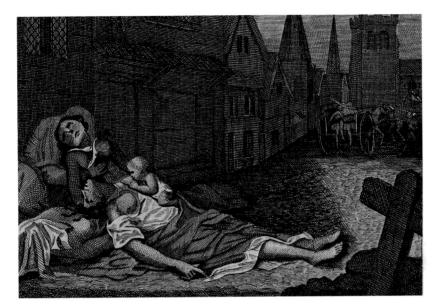

the victims once the initial plague pits had been filled. Citizens had to resort to burying their own children, and Agnolo di Tura "the Fat" had to bury his five children without help. Agnolo also noted that due to the rocky soil many graves were too shallow and the local dogs would dig up the bodies and eat them.

ABOVE During London's Great Plague of 1665 only the well-off had the chance to flee. The poorer citizens had to take their chances with the bubonic plague.

the victims once the initial plague pits had been filled. Citizens had to resort to burying their own children, and Agnolo di Tura "the Fat" had to bury his five children without help. Agnolo also noted that due to the rocky soil many graves were too shallow and the local dogs would dig up the bodies and eat them.

In Avignon, France, the presence of the Pope did not protect the population and it was recorded that 7,000 houses were boarded up and deserted and 11,000 corpses were buried in one graveyard in the first six weeks of the plague. It is estimated that 120,000 to 150,000 died in this area in the initial outbreak in 1348. So many needed burial in Avignon that the Pope blessed the Rhône River so that the multitude of corpses dumped into it would have a consecrated home.

When the plague hit England in 1347 to 1348, similar scenes were enacted, although it does not seem that there was a total breakdown in order. In Winchester, the church authorities insisted on burying the dead in consecrated ground within the cathedral precincts. They were determined to maintain this practice because the bishop, the holder of one of the most prestigious clerical positions in England, believed that on Judgment Day all good Christians would rise with the second coming of Christ, but only if they were buried in Church-sanctioned ground. The good citizens of Winchester were more concerned with the dangers to their physical health posed by the massed charnel pits in the center of town, rather than the spiritual health of the dead. Concerned citizens attacked several monks as they conducted burial ceremonies, and although the bishop threatened to excommunicate the perpetrators, he relented and new burial pits were consecrated beyond the city walls. Scenes

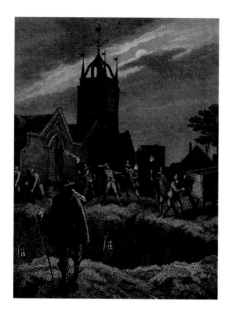

ABOVE **Churchyards rapidly filled with the dead. Adjoining land was consecrated and large pits were dug to ensure plague victims received a Christian burial.**

such as this were enacted throughout England where, due to the massed influx or corpses, consecrated land was in short supply. Village priests were reluctant to take church or manorial land for this purpose without written permission from local lords or bishops, but this was often not forthcoming because they were either dead or had fled. In most cases, land away from watercourses and towns was appropriated anyway. In London, new graveyards were opened at Smithfield and Spittle Croft. One of these had 50,000 bodies consigned to the earth. However, many smaller plague pits were opened with or without church approval.

The diarist Samuel Pepys (1633–1703) described how the authorities were overwhelmed by the plague of 1665 and tells of "The sad news of the death of so many in the parish of the plague, forty last night, the bell always going, either for deaths or burials." The death toll rises to such an extent that the living do not want to "carry the dead to be buried by daylight, the nights not sufficing to do it in."

In Pistoia, Italy, so numerous were the dead that church authorities were ordered not to ring bells during funerals lest it scare the inhabitants. The price of wax skyrocketed so much due to the many funerals being held that it was decreed that only two candles could be lit per funeral.

PERSECUTION OF THE JEWS

Apart from the obvious effects on society, such as economic dislocation and disenchantment with the Church, one violent outcome of the plague was the slaughter of thousands of Jews.

The Jews in England were lucky to avoid the burnings and hangings that erupted against their brethren across the Channel—not because the English were necessarily more tolerant and enlightened than other Europeans, but mainly because most Jews had been kicked out in 1290 by King Edward I. Those who remained lived within the community and enjoyed a low profile.

Not so for the European Jewish community. They had the misfortune of being a high-profile and unpopular minority within society who had one main economic activity: usury, or moneylending. In many jurisdictions ordinances had been passed limiting the economic opportunities of Jews. They were forbidden to hold military or civil positions, could not engage in a craft or agriculture, and weren't allowed to own land. That left them with one avenue toward wealth: usury, often at exorbitant rates. Despite these restrictions, the Jewish community had thrived during the 13th century as the economy and population throughout Europe expanded. However, by the time the plague reared its ugly head, a series of recessions and poor harvests, as well as the rise of large Christian banking houses, had reduced the moneylending activities of the Jews to small loans and pawnshops extorting high interest from the poor and the needy.

This economic imperative, coupled with superstitious fears of strange-looking people with different customs and languages, led to violent outbreaks throughout Europe, not rivaled until the holocaust under the Nazis.

The first attacks actually happened in the south of France in the spring of 1348 when the Christian communities of Narbonne and Carcassonne exterminated the entire Jewish population. The accusation that Jews were poisoning wells, causing the plague, fueled the hatred, and pogroms occurred across Europe over the next few years. Most of these massacres happened once the plague had hit town, but sometimes pogroms erupted before anybody had become sick. The Jewish communities in Antwerp and Brussels (in present-day Belgium) were entirely exterminated in 1350. There were almost no Jews left in Germany or the Low Countries by 1351.

While some authorities and rulers tried to stop the violence, most were complicit and some even encouraged it.

BELOW **It was reported that in 1349 the citizens of Strasbourg, France, set upon the Jewish community and burned them on huge pyres.**

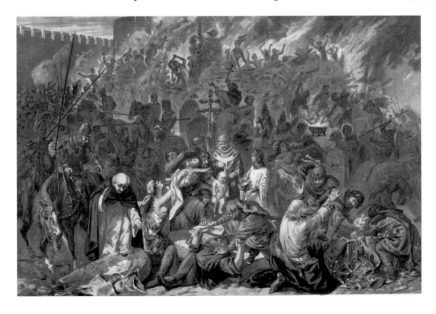

The papacy did not actively encourage the persecution, but its tacit acceptance and refusal to condemn the violent actions no doubt contributed to the death toll.

Why were people so easily convinced that there was a conspiracy to poison the water and that it was necessary to eliminate the Jews? It was considered that the plague was actually sent to punish the sinners, and what greater sin could there be to allow heretics to live among you? Many Jews were given the opportunity to convert to Christianity, and could have saved themselves if they followed this course. There was also a perception that the Jewish community was less affected by the plague and had a lower mortality rate. This may have been because of religious practices that encouraged a greater degree of hygiene than their neighbors enjoyed. These included frequent washing and rapid burial of the dead.

THE FLAGELLANTS

The Flagellants were an elitist organization chiefly drawn from the wealthier and better-educated classes. They were most prevalent in German-speaking lands and in the Low Countries. The inspiration of the movement was actually a letter supposedly delivered by an angel to the Church of St. Peter in Jerusalem around 1343. This besought good Christians to scourge themselves of the world's sins just as God was scourging the earth through the plague. By inflicting self-abuse, Flagellants believed that they could atone for mankind's sins and rid the world of the plague.

BELOW **The Flagellants were a short-lived response to the crisis brought about by the plague. They sought to show their devotion to God through suffering.**

Discouraged from acting in England, one large group did make it over the Channel where Sir Robert of Avesbury recorded their activities:

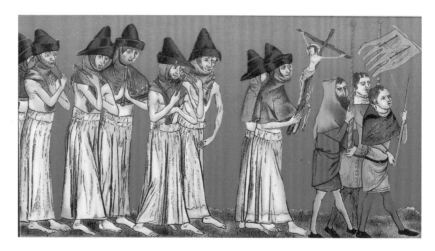

In that same year of 1349, about Michaelmas [September 29] over six hundred men came to London from Flanders, mostly of Zeeland and Holland origin. Sometimes at St Paul's and sometimes at other points in the city they made two daily public appearances wearing clothes from the thighs to the ankles, but otherwise stripped bare. Each wore a cap marked with a red cross in front and behind. Each had in his right hand a scourge with three tails. Each tail had a knot and through the middle of it there were sometimes sharp nails fixed. They marched naked in a file one behind the other and whipped themselves with these scourges on their naked and bleeding bodies. Four of them would chant in their native tongue, and another four would chant in response like a litany. Thrice they would all cast themselves on the ground in this sort of procession, stretching out their hands like the arms of a cross. The singing would go on and, the one who was in the rear of those thus prostrated acting first, each of them in turn would step over the others and give one stroke with his scourge to the man lying under him. This went on from the first to the last until each of them had observed the ritual to the full tale of those on the ground. Then each put on his customary garments and always wearing their caps and carrying their whips in their hands they retired to their lodgings. It is said that every night they performed the same penance.

—"THE FLAGELLANTS ATTEMPT TO REPEL THE BLACK DEATH, 1349," EYEWITNESS TO HISTORY, WWW.EYEWITNESSTOHISTORY.COM, 2010

It is unlikely that each individual could suffer the lacerations described above twice a day and usually from a group of penitents, only a small proportion would scarify themselves in a ceremony. Nevertheless, the Flagellants did put on quite a show.

THE PLAGUE TODAY

Despite the invention of penicillin, the plague is still a danger and isolated outbreaks are reported on a regular basis. Sydney, Australia, experienced an outbreak in 1900. The United States suffered several outbreaks in the 1970s and 1980s. In 1983, 40 people were infected and six died. The likely causes are skinning an infected prairie dog or handling a wild chipmunk.

Today, antibiotics rapidly cure any individual unfortunate enough to be diagnosed with the plague. There is also a vaccine that gives protection in hotspots around the world. Plague is still endemic in some areas of Africa, Eastern Europe, and Asia. The last mass infection reported was in the Indian state of Gujurat in 1994, where an outbreak of pneumonic plague caused scenes of confusion and panic. Mass use of antibiotics and vaccination nipped the outbreak in the bud.

CHAPTER 3

VENEREAL DISEASE

"ONE NIGHT WITH VENUS, AND A LIFETIME with Mercury." This delightful play on words hides the horrible reality of early venereal disease (VD) treatments. *Lues venerea* is the Latin term for venereal disease (sexually transmitted disease), derived from Venus the goddess of Love. Mercury here alludes to the toxic, heavy metal often used to cure these diseases. It could be injected up the urethra, rubbed on the sores as a lotion, or swallowed as a medicine. This often led to mercury poisoning, which frequently resulted in kidney failure and death. Only the invention of the first rubberized condom in 1855 gave humanity a reliable shield against these diseases.

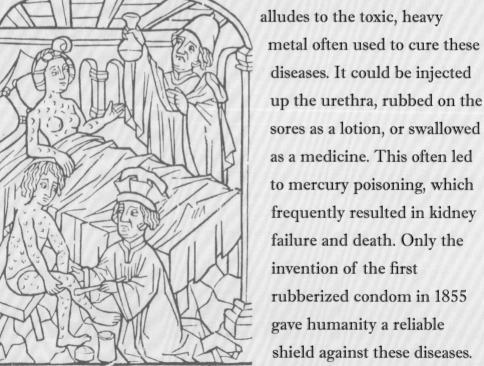

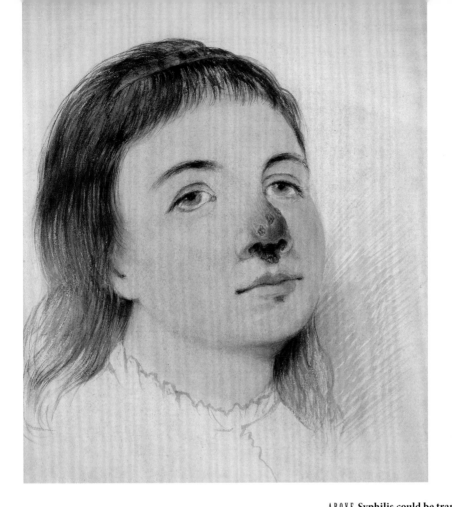

ABOVE Syphilis could be transmitted to infants in the womb. The first sign that a child was infected was often when the nasal cartilage began to rot.

SYPHILIS

The origin of syphilis is still something of a mystery, although it is most likely to have originated in the Americas and to have been taken to Europe by returning Spanish explorers who had engaged in sexual contact with the indigenous population. Alternatively, it may have been an existing pathogen that became more virulent and was previously confused with leprosy.

When syphilis was first recorded in Europe in 1495, its pustules often covered the body from head to foot and caused large gobbets of rotting flesh to fall from the victim's body—particularly the face—and led to death within a few months. This appalling new disease also gave rise to weeping pus-filled abscesses that ate away at the flesh and could penetrate into the bones. The illness first became epidemic in the French army; when the army dispersed after King Charles VIII's siege of Naples in 1495, the soldiers and their camp followers returned to their homelands taking the new pox with them.

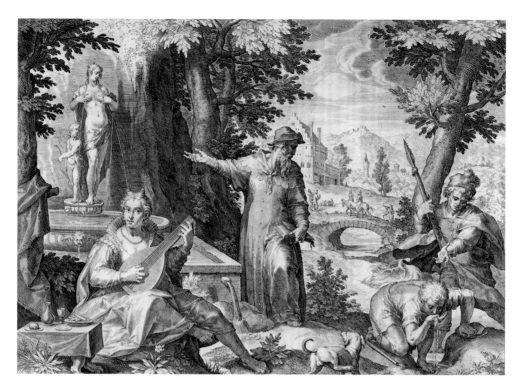

ABOVE **A 16th-century woodcut warning against the temptations of the flesh. A hunter and a shepherd are urged to resist wine, women, and song.**

Such was the disgust caused by this new disease that all nations sought to make their enemies responsible. The English and Germans called it the "French disease," while the French called it the "Naples pox." The Poles named it the "Russian disease," while for the Turks it was the "Christian disease." The Japanese called it the "Chinese Pox," while in India the Europeans were blamed for the "Portuguese disease." Two names stuck: "syphilis," named after a shepherd in an allegorical poem where the poor fellow gives in to sexual temptation and is infected, and the "great pox."

By 1546 the disease had evolved into its current form, where the primary stage is the appearance of genital sores that heal after several weeks. The secondary stage is characterized by rashes and flu-like symptoms, such as fever, lassitude, and aches and pains. The tertiary stage is where the causative bacterium, *Treponema pallidum*, really goes to work and begins to eat away at selected parts of the body. It can take many years for this stage to show externally, though in the meantime the host remains infectious and can transmit the disease to other people through sexual congress.

Once it moves out of its latent stage, the bacterium causes abscesses to crop up all over the body before it begins eating away at the digits, the face, the internal organs, and in particular, the brain. John Batman (1801–39), the founder of Melbourne,

Australia, is usually portrayed as a handsome and heroic explorer gazing over new and fertile lands. He should be portrayed with a scarf wrapped around his face to cover the hole where his nose was before it was eaten away with tertiary syphilis. His wife died a penniless and syphilis-raddled whore in Geelong. Syphilis can also infect the nervous system, leading to paralysis, insanity, and blindness. The father of the British politician Winston Churchill (1874–1965) died of this aspect of the infection, and Winston himself was fortunate that he was not affected in the womb, as there is some evidence that his mother was rather "loose" in her ways and may have picked up the infection. Many infants born to syphilitic mothers were infected and afflicted with deformities including blindness, deafness, and peg-shaped teeth. This disease effectively modified itself to ensure a successful career attacking humans and, if it were not for penicillin, it would still be a worldwide scourge today.

The chancres (sores) found around the genital region of sufferers are still the main way in which the disease is transmitted to new hosts. Approximately 12 million new cases are reported each year, but one shot of penicillin is normally enough to cure it; fortunately, no antibiotic-resistant strains have yet been found.

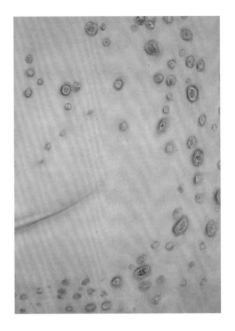

ABOVE **Tubercular syphilide erupted all over the skin in the later stage of the disease, the tubercles ranging in size from that of a pea to a hazelnut.**

BELOW **Syphilitic paronychia was caused by the bacteria eating away at the nail, the cuticle, and the flesh below.**

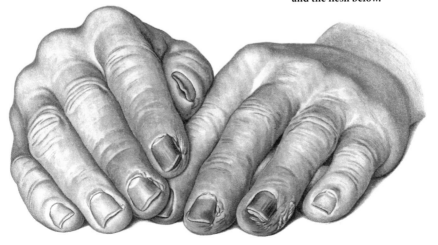

Sex and Disease

Syphilis is of course not the only sexually transmitted disease to rely on humans for its survival. The most ancient scourges such as herpes, and the latest illnesses such as AIDS, are able to thrive in the human biome due to our uniquely broad sexual practices. Most animals have short and seasonal bursts of sexual activity that usually involves genital-to-genital contact. Humans' predilection for anal, oral, vaginal, and penile sex that continues throughout adult life and does not have only reproductive functions, means there are a plethora of mucous membranes, body fluids, skin lesions, mouths, and orifices through which cunning microbes can enter a new host.

Herpes was probably inherited in its oral form from our primate ancestors, but has now mutated within humans to a genital form. This is also the case with genital warts, which were first described by the ancient Greeks. These most often form around the area where sexual contact has taken place: under the foreskin, around the anus, or surrounding the labia. These are particularly nasty warts and rather than being flat or bulbous like normal skin warts, genital warts form fleshy protuberances or "figs" as the ancient Romans referred to them.

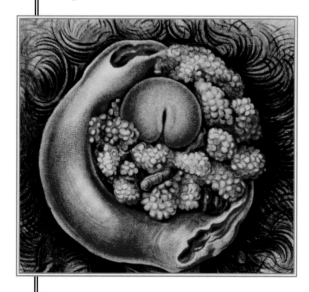

LEFT A severe case of genital warts in a male patient. The ancient Romans referred to these as "figs" because of their appearance.

GONORRHEA

Gonorrhea has developed a unique symbiosis with mankind and has no other animal reservoir. The bacterium *Neisseria gonorrhoeae* lives in the urinary tract, a hostile environment in which few other pathogens can live. Sores and pustules are characteristic symptoms of this disease, along with noxious emissions. Men experience burning as they urinate, but women often have no symptoms whatsoever. There are two accepted versions of why it is called "the clap." One is that it came from the root word *clapier*, French for brothel. The other possible derivation comes from the early treatment where the offending male member was "clapped" between two hands to expel any noxious fluids.

In the West, gonorrhea was first recognized by an Act of the English Parliament in 1161 seeking to limit its spread, while Louis IX in France passed a decree in 1256 calling on sufferers to be exiled. Crusaders in the Middle East noticed its prevalence among the local population.

The early treatments were painful affairs and involved injecting various substances up the middle of the penis with syringes. Mercury, silver nitrate, and even pepper were forced up the urethra in an effort to cure the nasty little bug.

Though these remedies were occasionally useful and would at least treat the symptoms, they rarely cleared the bacterium out of the system. It was not until the advent of antibiotics that a true cure was found. However, as early as 1983 an outbreak in North Carolina demonstrated that some strains of gonorrhea are developing resistance to penicillin.

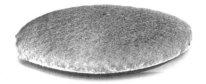
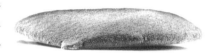

ABOVE The *Neisseria gonorrhoeae* bacterium, shown in this scanning electron micrograph, is one of the toughest bacteria around.

BELOW Lesions such as these often develop on the skin of gonorrhea sufferers. However, some infected people display no symptoms at all.

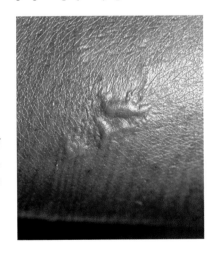

THE BACTERIUM *NEISSERIA GONORRHOEAE* LIVES IN THE URINARY TRACT, A HOSTILE ENVIRONMENT IN WHICH FEW OTHER PATHOGENS CAN LIVE. SORES AND PUSTULES ARE CHARACTERISTIC SYMPTOMS OF THIS DISEASE, ALONG WITH NOXIOUS EMISSIONS.

SKIN BREEDERS

SEXUALLY transmitted diseases (STDs) occur when humans mate. These infections occur when insects mate in us!

1 BOTFLY: Humans in Central America and Africa may receive a painful bite from a fly. Soon the bite grows and something inside begins to wiggle: this is a botfly larva (pictured below) growing to maturity under the skin.

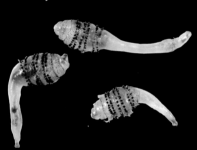

2 JIGGERS: Native to South America, these nasty little sand fleas (pictured left) have colonized most of sub-Saharan Africa. A female jigger burrows into the sole of the host's foot and proceeds to lay several eggs. These then reproduce under the skin, leading to large patches of dead, soft tissue and open, weeping sores. Each jigger has to be removed individually. If untreated, the infestation can lead to gangrene and eventual amputation.

3 SCABIES: This comes from a mite called *Sarcoptes scabiei* (pictured below). It burrows into the top layer of the skin and lays three eggs a day. These eggs hatch and travel back to the surface, causing dreadful itching. Untreated, this can develop into the "Norwegian Itch," a crusty hive of parasites forming leather-like skin on the host (see page 216).

LEFT If it is untreated, scabies can lead to a crusty build-up of dead flesh filled with millions of tiny parasites. Even today it is difficult to get rid of.

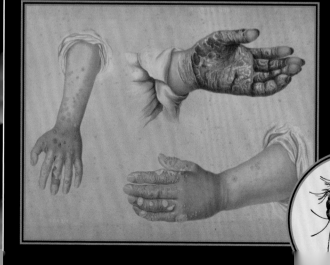

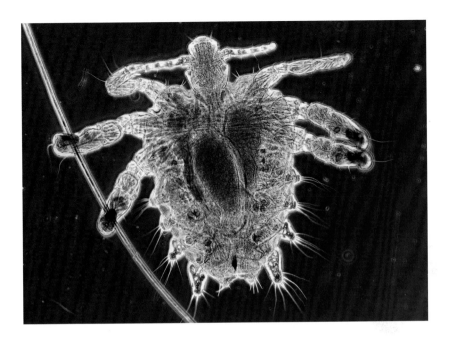

CRABS

Chimpanzees only have head lice (genus *Pediculus*), while gorillas are blessed with pubic lice (genus *Phthirus*) or "crabs." Humans have both: head lice and pubic lice. While it's likely that different hair lice strains evolved with the human–chimp divergence 6 million years ago, DNA studies indicate that early hominids picked up crabs from gorilla populations 3 million years ago. Whether this was from cross-species sexual contact, predation, or cohabitation in the same environment is unknown.

Pubic lice are named "crabs" due to their strong resemblance to this crustacean. Having evolved to move between widely separated pubic hairs, their legs stick out from their body, allowing them to crawl quickly around their environment. They are usually transmitted through sexual congress, and can survive on unwashed linen for up to two days. Their only food source is human blood. They feed by biting the skin at the base of the pubic hair follicles. The anticoagulant transmitted in their bite leads to itching and inflammation.

As they have been present for much of human history, a large number of remedies have been tried. A liberal application of viper juice, or bacon grease mixed with ashes, were two suggested cures. Today topical creams are available to kill these nasty little critters. However, hair lice are developing resistance to most common treatments: hopefully the same will not happen with their pubic cousins.

THE CONDOM IN HISTORY

There is scant evidence for the use of the condom in the archaeological record. The earliest reference to their use in history may stem from Minoan society (1500 BCE) where a myth details how King Minos sought to protect his wife from infection by serpents and scorpions contained within his sperm by using a goat's bladder as a prophylactic. Various kinds of animal gut including sheep intestines were used in classical times. In ancient China "glans" condoms of silk or skin were used. These only covered the tip or glans of the penis and must have been difficult to keep in place.

The oldest preserved condoms were discovered in an archaeological dig in Dudley Castle near Birmingham in England. Dated to approximately 1642, they were made of cattle, sheep, and fish intestines. Charles II was engaged there in the Civil War against his Parliamentarian foe. He needed to ensure that prophylactics were issued to his troops, as many were falling prey, not to Parliamentarian bullets or round shot, but to syphilis.

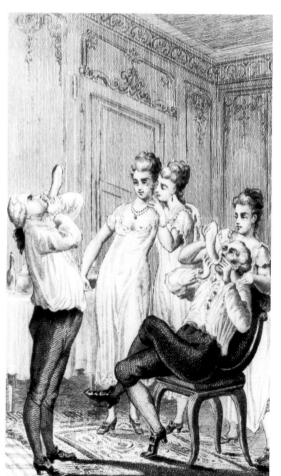

By the 18th century new technologies allowed condoms to be produced *en masse*. They were available in a range of qualities and sizes and were made of bladders or intestines softened with sulfur and lye. Also available were versions made from linen treated with various chemicals.

While the Venetian author Casanova is renowned for his lovemaking, he was also engaged in quality control: He would blow up each condom like a balloon before use, just to check that there were no leaks.

No such testing would have been required for the excellent product offered by Mrs. Phillips in her shop in Leicester Square, London, during the 1700s. These were no doubt the most spectacular form

LEFT **The notorious womanizer Giacomo Casanova (1725–98) testing a condom by filling it with air.**

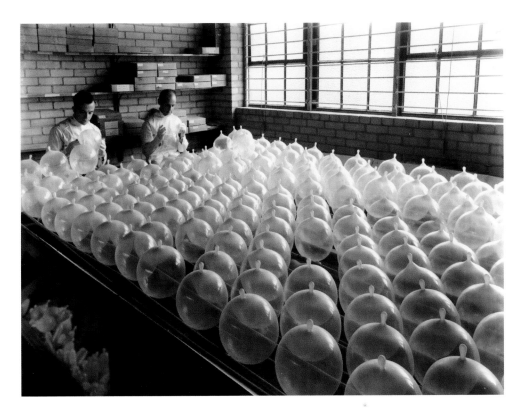

ABOVE Testing condoms, 1930s. Vulcanized rubber and latex condoms were rigorously checked before leaving the factory.

of the condom in history. Each condom was 8 inches (20 cm) of goat intestine, pickled, scented, and individually shaped on glass molds by Mrs. Phillips and her comely daughters. Each condom was secured around the base with a ribbon. These could either be colored with the red, white, and blue of the Union Jack, or with a gentleman's regimental colors. These top-of-the-line articles were named *baudruches superfines*. She also advertised her *superfine double* in *The Tatler* in 1709. This line was for the more cautious gentleman and included two superimposed sheaths of sheep gut.

Charles Goodyear (1800–60) invented the process of rubber vulcanization in 1839. The first rubber condoms were produced in 1855. One of the "advantages" of these early condoms was that they could be washed and reused several times.

In the 1920s latex was invented, and this allowed the production of the strong but flexible condoms that are used today. Black, red, ribbed, multicolored, aloe vera, banana- or strawberry-flavored, the variety of condoms now available has advanced considerably from the early days of the sheep gut.

4

SHOCKING SURGERY

THE EARLIEST KNOWN SURGICAL PROCEDURE is trephination (or trepanation). This involves boring or scraping a hole in the skull without damaging the underlying tissues. The first instance of this in the archaeological records is an assemblage of skulls from burial sites in France dated to approximately 6500 BCE. The percentage of skulls found shows that it was a common procedure, whether to release "evil spirits" or repair impacted craniums is not known. Many of the trepanned wounds were healed, demonstrating a successful surgical outcome. In human history this has not always been the case, and many "shocking surgeries" have led to misery and death. Two developments turned the odds in favor of the patient: anesthesia and disinfectant.

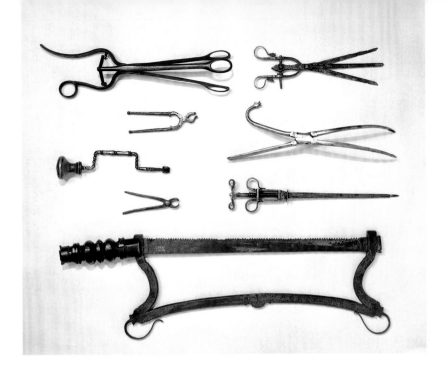

SURGEONS

In the early days of medicine, surgeons were not the exalted persons they are today, or even in Victorian times. A surgeon was of a lower order both in the medical profession and in the social hierarchy. Often called "sawbones," they were not trained as doctors in philosophy or theology. Medical men who described themselves as surgeons were considered to be little better than manual workers. Their medical training, if they had any, was limited. They possessed some knowledge of anatomy and could cut off things, cut out things, set broken limbs, treat venereal disease, help with childbirth and, if particularly ambitious, try a little trepanning or stone removal.

They used a surgeon's kit of knives, saws, needles, forceps, and scalpels to carry out their physical carpentry. They were, like the rest of the medical profession, unversed in the concept of hygiene and rarely cleaned their instruments or operating tables. The first operations with anesthetic were not carried out until 1846. Surgeons would operate on patients while still in their street clothes; and they often kept silk ligatures in bunches threaded through their buttonholes or tucked into a pocket. Any operation was hazardous in the extreme for the patient, and surgical wards had a terrible stench caused by gangrene and rotting flesh. Patients who survived the shock of going under the knife had a zinc tray placed under their wounds to catch the "laudable pus" that seeped from the wound and was seen as a good sign.

ABOVE This array of lethal-looking surgical instruments dates from the 16th and 17th centuries. They were utilized to remove teeth, bullets, arrows, bladder stones, and limbs.

AMPUTATIONS

The advent of massed gunpowder weapons (post 1500) saw the maiming of thousands of limbs due to shot wounds. A lead shot from these early weapons flattened on impact, leading to ghastly injuries, most of which featured shattered bones and joints. Surgeons needed to develop a new skill. Rather than the delicate process of removing arrowheads or sewing sword wounds, they had to become proficient at amputation.

This was a brutal business. The surgeon first used a sharpened knife (no scalpels then) and cut away the flesh where the amputation was to be made. Rounded knives like scythes were preferred, and with a quick twist of the wrist the flesh could be severed right around the bone.

Standing next to the surgeon would be a brazier with red-hot irons, which he would use to seal the arteries and prevent blood loss. Then he would cut the bone off using a razor-sharp saw. On the brazier was a pot of boiling oil. Once the amputation was made, the surgeon poured this oil over the bloodied stump to cauterize the wound. Any surviving nerve endings would make the pain intolerable, and many patients died on the table from shock and pain. If boiling oil was not available, gunpowder was poured over the wound and ignited—hardly a

BELOW German soldiers are treated for combat wounds in the 16th century. The patient on the left is having his lower leg sawn off. The flesh had to be sliced off first.

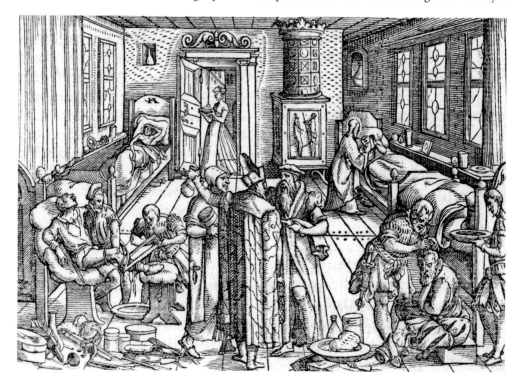

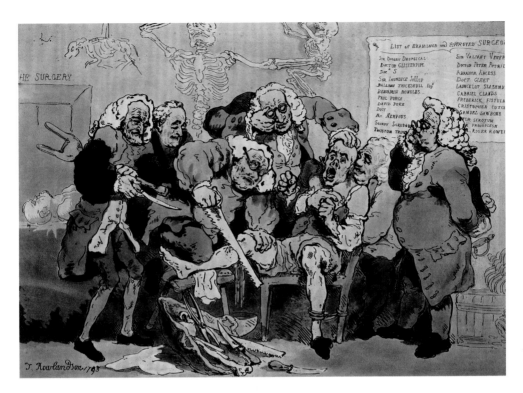

more pleasant option. Another possibility was to use a cautery knife. This was a sharp blade that was heated until it was red-hot. As it cut through the patient's flesh it also cauterized the wound, particularly the smaller blood vessels.

Even those who survived this treatment spent days in agony as the wound slowly healed, if it did at all. Observers in the 16th century noticed patients in military hospitals running high fevers with swollen, pus-filled, red wounds.

ABOVE Six surgeons are participating in this 18th-century amputation. The patient is unsedated and obliged to watch the whole procedure. The surgeon on the left holds a cautery knife.

Amputation Innovator

Ambroise Paré (1510–90) was a French military surgeon who brought an unusual degree of compassion to his trade, and would only operate when absolutely necessary. Despite this, he is considered the father of modern-day surgery. Among many innovations, Paré stopped the practice of castrating patients who were due to go under the knife to treat hernias. Most importantly for the subject at hand, during a campaign to capture Turin, Italy, in 1537, Paré painted the wounds of amputated limbs with a styptic to stop the bleeding—a mixture of egg yolk, turpentine, and rose oil—when he ran out of the customary hot oil. An improvement was immediately noticed: Paré's patients rested well and their wounds healed. However, he was not entirely satisfied

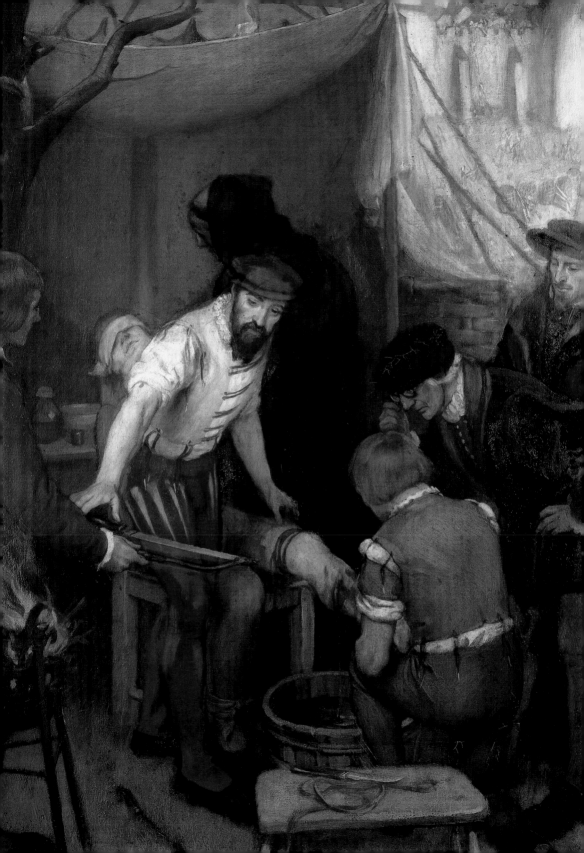

with his styptic and, like any good medical practitioner today, he tried to find an improved recipe. He bribed a successful Turin surgeon for his formula and after two years managed to extract the recipe: just-whelped puppies were to be fried in lily oil along with earthworms soaked in turpentine—a blend of science and superstition.

In 1552, during a siege, Paré used silk or twine to act as a ligature to control bleeding from arteries. He had noted that cauterized arteries took a long time to heal, causing fever and pain. In his estimation only two out of five patients were likely to survive this procedure. As the wound healed, the scab fell off and another cauterization was required, eating up "a great quantity of flesh and other nervous parts." A side effect of this creeping cauterization was that long pieces of exposed bone remained sticking out of the flesh once it had healed.

Recognized as a genius, Paré was royal physician to four kings of France. After his pioneering work, styptics became commonly used and surgeons believed that the concoctions would reduce bleeding as well as stop infection. Turpentine was a common ingredient, as were alum and vitriol. By the 1670s, some surgeons believed so strongly in the virtues of styptics that a ligature was deemed superfluous. A practitioner in 1670s Paris, Dr. Rabel, so strongly believed in his styptic "vulnerary water" that he arranged a demonstration in front of Louis XIV's war minister at the Hôtel des Invalides. He amputated the thigh of a soldier and closed the wound using only his styptic and bandages to stem the bleeding. But no matter how much of the styptic was painted on, the soldier bled out in front of the gathered audience.

LEFT **Ambroise Paré was considerate toward his patients. He utilized ligatures to control bleeding rather than painful and dangerous cauterization with gunpowder.**

The Tourniquet and Other Improvements

The next major development in the art of amputation was the invention of the tourniquet in 1674. This allowed the upper limb to be tightly bound, stemming blood flow into the lower limb and reducing the need for cauterization.

In the early 18th century, Jean Louis Petit improved upon this method by introducing the screw tourniquet. This allowed the veins to be compressed in an adjustable manner. Strictly speaking, neither the ligature nor the tourniquet were recent inventions, as both ancient Greek and Roman surgeons had used these techniques. Cautery did not stop the flow of blood from the thigh, due to the width of the arteries. The tourniquet allowed amputations to take place as high as the hips or shoulder, ensuring any diseased flesh was cut away.

BELOW **This sophisticated tourniquet, developed by Petit in 1718, allowed the surgeon to vary the pressure applied to the arteries. The pad would be placed where the most pressure was needed.**

Nevertheless these "chop" amputations, where the bone and the flesh were all cut at the same place, led to bloody exposed wounds so that even when they had healed it was near impossible to attach a prosthetic limb to the damaged skin. In 1679 James Yonge of Plymouth, England, solved this problem when he invented the "flap" amputation; in this method skin was preserved on one side of the amputation and was then folded and stitched over the wound.

The final improvement in the technique of amputation was the replacement of the silk or linen ligature with catgut; instead of causing inflammation and infection within the wound, it was naturally absorbed by the body.

The First Ambulance

Dominique-Jean Larrey (1766–1842) began his career as a surgeon in the French navy, but was unsuited to this career as he suffered from seasickness. He was reassigned to the army and saw that field hospitals were too far behind the front lines to render aid to wounded soldiers on time. Soldiers were loaded onto slow carts and transported at least 3 miles (5 km) behind the lines, where clogged roads often meant that they died before reaching the hospital.

He designed a speedy two-wheeled cart—"the flying ambulance." Organized into columns of up to 20 ambulances, they were purpose-built carts pulled by two horses. The enclosed body protected the patients from the elements. Crewed with specialist medical personnel, doctors, and quartermasters, protected by an infantry escort, and equipped with bandages and opiates, they transported the wounded straight from the battlefield, even in the heat of the action. During Napoleon's Egyptian campaign of 1798 Larrey used camels instead.

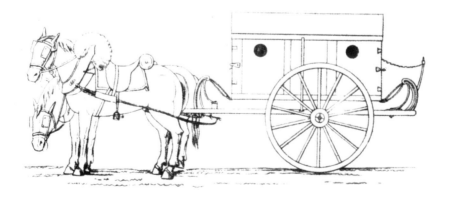

REJUVENATION BY GRAFTING

Dr. Serge Voronoff was a Russian-born surgeon who was Director of Experimental Surgery at the Collège de France in Paris during the 1920s and 1930s. While he made excellent surgical innovations, he also made some big mistakes.

While visiting Cairo in 1898, Voronoff was able to observe some eunuchs who had been castrated at about 4 or 5 years old. He noted disparagingly that they had many negative health outcomes from this cruel procedure. They were overweight, with enlarged pelvises and breasts; they had smooth, droopy, and hairless faces, and displayed a marked lack of energy and a flabby, toneless musculature. They seemed to be prematurely aged, lacked enterprise, and had poor memories.

Voronoff ascribed the symptoms to lack of testicles, and after 18 years mulling on the problem he came up with the crackpot scheme to somehow replace worn-out testicles on older French men with young, active testicles, so that they could regain their youthful virility. Despite the agony that he put his patients through, many more men volunteered to get the treatment than he could possibly service. The doctor practiced his technique on animals before trying it on humans.

An ape and a man were placed side by side on two hospital gurneys and knocked out with a combination of ethyl chloride and chloroform. During the 1930s chloroform was still a commonly used anesthetic and people would even get together for chloroform parties, little realizing the damage the drug was doing to their livers, kidneys, and hearts. It is not used as an anesthetic today due to the side effects it can cause. Once they were unconscious, their scrotums and upper thighs were shaved and painted with iodine. The monkey then had his

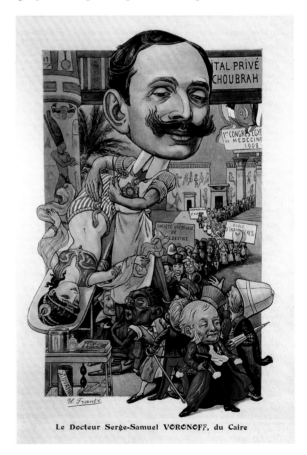

Le Docteur Serge-Samuel VORONOFF, du Caire

RIGHT Voronoff was infamous for grafting slivers of monkey testicles onto men's gonads. Here, he is portrayed performing an appendectomy.

scrotum sliced open and one of his testicles surgically removed before it was placed onto a sterile surface and cut with a scalpel into six thin slices.

While this procedure was going on, the male human patient had his scrotum sliced open and his testicle popped out of the ball sac, although it was still attached to his groin. A fine grater was used to scarify (roughen) the exposed testicle. Three of the slices of monkey testicle were then laid against the man's bloodied testicle and it was hoped that the two types of testicular material would bond together as the patient's testicle healed. The several layers of the scrotum were then stitched up and the same procedure was carried out on the other testicle. This delicate procedure required a great deal of expertise.

Voronoff was lauded by the medical establishment and wrote a book on his procedure called *Rejuvenation by Grafting*. The book had many case studies and even included before and after photos. He also claimed that the sex drive of his patients had increased, and that they had better memories, a stronger work ethic, and even improved eyesight, so that they could dispense with their glasses. He even proposed that some forms of dementia and schizophrenia would be healed by the procedure. No doubt the book did not include the information that his first two operations had

BELOW **These before (left) and after (right) pictures show a man who has benefited from Voronoff's treatment.**

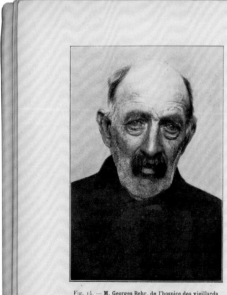

Fig. 14. — **M. Georges Behr, de l'hospice des vieillards de Douera, âgé de 73 ans, en 1924.**
Avant la greffe.

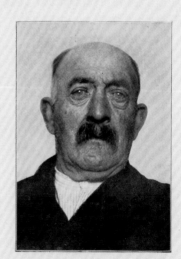

Fig. 15. — **M. Georges Behr, âgé de 74 ans, en 1925.**
Un an après la greffe.

almost killed the subjects and that the grafts had to be removed to avoid blood poisoning. The American John R. Brinkley adopted Voronoff's procedure and would perform at least 50 operations a week in his home state of Kansas. For some reason it was decided that prisoners in San Quentin State Prison would benefit from the procedure and at least 300 had monkey implants placed into their testicles.

A wave of testicle grafting swept the world. In the years between 1920 and 1940, more than 45 surgeons utilised Voronoff's techniques to conduct more than 2,000 xenotransplants from non-human to human primates in many countries around the world. This included more than 500 men from France, while others subjected themselves to the procedure in the United States, Italy, Russia, Brazil, Chile, and India. Positive reports poured in and it was decided that a follow-up dose of monkey testicle was even more effective. Re-transplantation became common. Voronoff held that this second graft, which in half the cases was done five or six years after the first, attained positive results similar to those recorded in the original surgery. Hopefully for these poor men it was more than merely a placebo effect.

By the 1940s clinical tests proved that the immune system of recipients would neutralize and then destroy any implants, absorbing and dissolving the intrusive flesh. Despite this setback, Voronoff married a woman 25 years his junior and they had a loving, happy relationship for many years.

CASTRATION

One of the most difficult operations for any man to live through is castration, or gelding. Persian, Roman, Greek, North African, Chinese, and Indian rulers all employed eunuchs in a variety of roles including spying, the civil service, and guarding harems, something they were particularly suited for. They were also used as entertainers. Until comparatively recently it was seen as indecent for women to appear on stage, and when a high note had to be reached it was the castrato who donned the goddess's costume and rang out a melody. The practice of using emasculated children to sing in the Vatican court was only stopped in 1878.

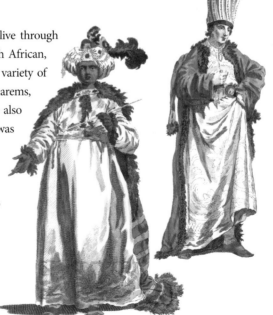

RIGHT **Eunuchs were trusted members of many courts. These figures, painted in 1749, were in charge of a harem.**

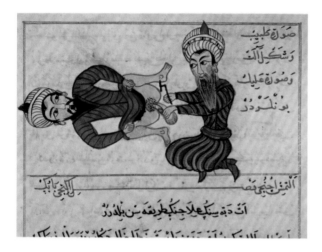

LEFT **The act of gonadectomy required a firm hand and a steely nerve. A willing subject may have been harder to find.**

The health effects of castration (gonadectomy) were not all bad. Those who were castrated before the onset of puberty retained their high voice, slight build, lack of pubic and facial hair, small genitalia, and rarely developed a sex drive. Some became practiced in sexual acts and were professional catamites. Due to a lack of sexual hormones that retard long bone growth in late puberty, they were often quite tall. Muscle mass and body strength often decreased along with bone density, and body fat often migrated to the hips, buttocks, and chest. Male-pattern baldness never struck a castrated man, although hair did not grow back if he was bald before the procedure. Those who lost their penis (penectomy) as well as their testicles were often subject to urinary incontinence. Eunuchs often lived 14 to 19 years longer than other men from similar socioeconomic backgrounds. Why they lived longer is not known, but it could perhaps be attributed to not always thinking about sex, chasing sex, or procreating, leading to a less stressful lifestyle. Modern eunuchs have a reduced incidence of diabetes and heart disease.

Eunuchs in China

At one stage up to 10,000 eunuchs lived in the Forbidden City in Beijing, where they formed the administrative center of the Manchu Empire. It was said that at night in the imperial palace there would be thousands of men and women, but only one pair of testicles; these belonged to the emperor. Eunuchs were the only ones trusted to manage the imperial harem and to come near the emperor, as it was less likely that they would endanger him.

How Chinese men became gelded was no laughing matter. Select dynasties of practitioners who had carried out this practice for thousands of years were the only people licensed to emasculate individuals. The mortality rate was estimated at 2 out of 100, which speaks volumes for the expertise of these families. Many men volunteered to be castrated as a means to escape the grinding poverty of Imperial China, although they needed a member of the Confucian civil service to vouch for their character. Many young boys were sold by their families, and after the operation they were drafted into the palace where they were favored by young ladies in the harem.

So many males would not have been volunteered for the blade, if there had not been a good chance of success. The "knifers," as they were known, received six *taels* of silver for each successful operation. They also had to nurse their patients through the initial phase of recovery.

The procedure took place just beyond the walls of the Forbidden City. The patient reclined on a low bed and was asked, once more, if he would regret being castrated. If "no" was the reply, he was pinned to the bed and two men separated and firmly held down his legs. Tight bandages were wrapped around the patient's thighs and waist before an opium-laced tea was administered to him. The last sensation his penis and testicles would ever feel was when they were washed with Szechuan pepper water to desensitize them.

Once these preparations were complete, the knifer took a razor-sharp blade, grabbed the penis and testicles, and cut them all off, as close to the pubic area as possible. A metal plug was then inserted into the urethra, and the wound was covered with a water-soaked cloth before being bandaged. The newly graduated eunuch was then made to walk around the operating room for two or three hours, supported by the surgeon's assistants, before finally being allowed to lie down.

He was not allowed to drink any liquid for three days, and the agony of the proto-eunuchs must have been extreme as their bladder filled and the wound healed. At the end of three days the bandages were removed and the plug was pulled out. The bladder would by this time be incredibly full, so hopefully the poor man would be able to relieve himself; if so, it was considered that the operation had been a success. If the plug hadn't worked and the urethra had become inflamed and infected, making the eunuch unable to urinate, a slow and painful death ensued. For those fortunate to survive, after three months their training would begin in princely establishments and, if approved by experienced eunuchs, they could be given a position in the imperial palace.

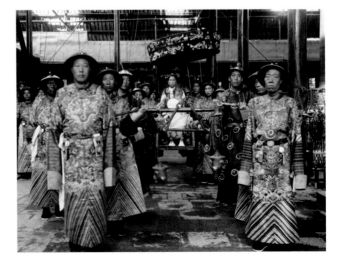

RIGHT **The Qing Dynasty employed thousands of eunuchs in the Forbidden City. The only male with testicles who was allowed to stay overnight was the emperor.**

KIDNEY AND BLADDER STONES

Greek mythology explains how Pandora's Box was opened to spread diseases and pests to plague mankind. There is no doubt that (if Pandora really existed) stones that inhabit the kidney and bladder are among the worst conditions she inflicted upon human beings. Throughout history these nasty growths have caused untold misery and pain. Some of the earliest medical procedures were developed to cure this scourge.

Kidney stones are caused by a range of factors and in particular arise when some people, particularly men, do not drink enough water. They are viscous-looking growths made up of sharp, angular edges with a pitted surface. They can grow to the size of a golf ball and usually remain unnoticed until they pass into the ureter on the way to the bladder. Here they become an entirely different beast and cause untold suffering. An inability to urinate combined with a constant urge to do so escalates into severe pain in the side, vomiting, nausea, blood and pus in the urine, and a ripping, burning sensation throughout the urinary tract.

Bladder stones are the diabolical twin of kidney stones. A buildup of minerals often caused by the bladder not emptying properly, they, too, are mainly found in men. Dante's Inferno could well have an entire level dedicated to men going through the unimaginable agony of passing a stone.

The First Transplants

John Hunter was a young surgeon growing up in Georgian London. During the 1760s he witnessed many tooth transplants. While most failed, with horrible repercussions for the patient, enough stuck to inform his fascinations with the "living principle." Surely, he thought, something living could be attached through surgical means to something else living. Chickens were used to prove his theories. A cockerel's testes were implanted within a hen. The spur of a cockerel was grafted to its head, and one lucky cockerel received a human tooth implanted into its comb! Of course most transplants were rejected, but the genetic similarity in Hunter's flock of chickens ensured that a significant number took. The first step toward skin grafting and organ transplants had been taken.

Stone Removal Through the Ages

In many periods of history, water was seen as dangerous and alcohol was the most common beverage. This led to dehydration, which exacerbated the development of this complaint. For some reason, males are more likely to be affected. Different societies have had different means of dealing with the problem, but they all involve cutting near the groin and anus.

Aulus Cornelius Celsus (ca. 25 BCE–ca. 50 CE) was an encyclopedist who gathered all known medical knowledge and practice from the ancient Greeks through to the Romans and wrote it down in his work *De Medicina*.

As recorded in *The Illustrated History of Surgery*, by Knut Haeger, Celsus described in glorious detail how to extract stones with the fingertips. First the patient was held down, with his legs held apart by two strong men. His knees were drawn as wide as possible. The doctor would carefully cut his nails and lubricate his left hand, and then he would insert two of his fingers, one after the other slowly into the patient's rectum. At the same time he would apply the fingers of his right hand to the lower abdomen. He did this with caution to avoid harming the bladder, in case his fingers should meet with the stone too strongly from both sides. (It was noted that lesions of the bladder could cause convulsions, which in turn could prove fatal.)

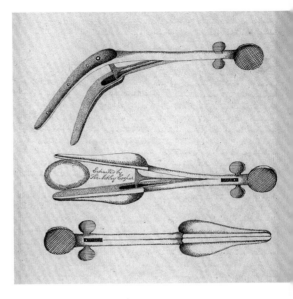

ABOVE Instruments were designed to penetrate the bladder and grind up or crush painful stones. Surgeons rarely sterilized them.

The stone was first sought out in the bladder neck and, if found there, it could be extracted with little trouble. If the stone was not located there or had receded, the doctor would push the fingers of his left hand up towards the upper part of the bladder, followed by the fingers of his right hand. With this two-handed method it was said that the stone could not avoid being found and would then be brought down the bladder neck.

Once the stone had descended thus far a crescent-shaped incision would be made in the skin near the anus, going into the bladder neck, with its corners slightly orientated toward the posterior pelvic bone. Then a transverse cut was made and the stone was extracted.

Cutting so close to the anus and urethra often led to fistulas. These are particularly nasty wounds that often link the anal canal with the bladder. (Women who undergo difficult deliveries can often develop them between the rectum and the vagina.)

This procedure which involved finding the stones by pushing the fingers up the anus and feeling through the intestinal wall to locate the stone before cutting into the perineum (the region between the genitals and anus) to remove the stones was the most common treatment in classical and medieval times.

In the years between 1500 and modern times there were many variations on this basic operation, which is now known as lithotomy. Some involved going through the urethra with a sharp blade to widen it and allow the stone to pop out, while others involved cutting above the pubic bone for access directly into the bladder. Of course, without proper antiseptics, many died of infection. Other side effects were almost as dire. Incontinence, fistulas, and impotence are regularly described. Perhaps the worst outcome was suffered by Samuel Pepys, the great London diarist. Although the surgery successfully removed the stones, he spent the last years of his life with a gaping wound just behind his scrotum that never healed.

As usual there were crank medicines designed to cure the condition, the most popular being the consumption of ground bees and snail shells mixed into broth and taken first thing in the morning. It was not until the 1822 invention of the lithotrite by Jean Zuléma Amussat (1796–1856) that a safer method was available. This did not require invasive surgery but involved passing a pair tongs up the urethra into the bladder, where they gripped the stone and ground it up through lever action. This device was improved upon by Jean Civiale (1792–1867), who performed his first successful lithotripsy with his trilabium, a device that gripped the stone in three claws while it was drilled into pieces. Once the stones were ground, they passed painlessly with urine.

While these procedures were a great improvement on previous methods, there were often post-procedural complications such as fever and infection. This problem was solved by the great British urologist Sir Henry Thompson. When he removed several stones from King Leopold I of Belgium in 1862, he sterilized his lithotrite. Previous practitioners had failed to clean their instruments between patients. The grateful king gave the surgeon £4,000 for his trouble. The crushed stones may still be seen at the Hunterian Museum in London.

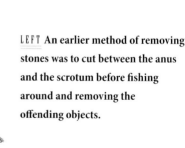

LEFT **An earlier method of removing stones was to cut between the anus and the scrotum before fishing around and removing the offending objects.**

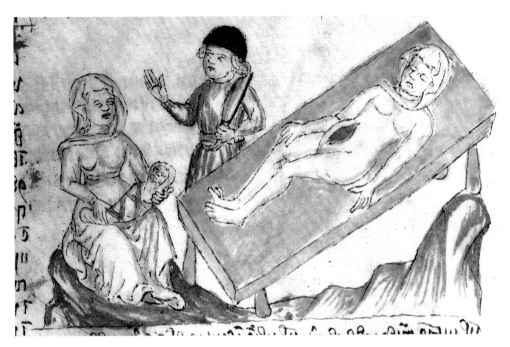

CESAREAN SECTION

Cesarean births are not a recent phenomenon; myths and legends abound. The young Buddha was born out of "his mother's right side." Dionysus, the Greek god of wine, was born by cesarean section two months premature, and Asclepius, the Greek god of medicine, was cut out of his mother's dead body. As early as the 7th century BCE, the Roman king Numa Pompilius (715–673 BCE) decreed that if a pregnant woman died the infant was to be removed by incision.

Recently deceased women didn't always need surgery to give birth; historical accounts abound where babies have been spontaneously ejected. The Spanish Inquisition hanged a heretic in 1551 and soon after, her fetus fell onto the gallows platform. In 1820, Cologne city council in Germany passed a law forbidding the practice of stuffing a dead woman's mouth with cloth, lest the fetus suffocate. Priests in the Catholic Church could be excommunicated if they buried a pregnant woman without a cesarean section being carried out to see if the child was alive. The priest had to be present to verify the condition of the child.

This procedure may have been named after Julius Caesar who was reputedly cut from his mother Aurelia's womb. She went on to enjoy a long and healthy life after founding a long line of emperors.

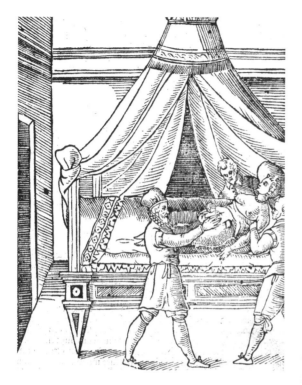

ABOVE **Despite some medical advances, cesarean births remained dangerous for the mother right up until the invention of antiseptics.**

The first recorded successful cesarean section on a living woman was performed by a pig farmer and animal castrator who lived in the German village of Sigershaufen around 1500. His wife was having difficulty giving birth and 13 midwives could not help her. He decided to take matters into his own hands and, using his knowledge gained in animal husbandry, he cut open his wife, extracted the child, and sewed up the uterus and abdominal wall.

In 1596 the first textbook on obstetrics, *La Commare o raccoglitrice* (The Book of Midwifery), was published in Venice, and became the standard work on the subject through 20 editions until 1713. Its chapter on cesarean births detailed how four assistants were required to hold down the pregnant woman, where to make the incision, and how to close the wound, wrap bandages, and apply an unguent of sour wine, roses, balsam, and healing herbs.

Nevertheless, until the 1870s women feared the operation with good reason. Poor hygiene led to a high percentage of deaths from the operation, usually involving peritonitis. It was not until 1882 that surgical sutures were used to sew up the uterus by German obstetricians Adolf Kehrer and Max Sänger. Also at this time it was recognized that removal of the womb at the same time could restrict bleeding; the first cesarean hysterectomy in the United States was performed in 1881.

LISTON AND THE RISE OF ANESTHESIA

The record as the most egotistical and dangerous surgeon might go to the Scottish practitioner Robert Liston (1794–1847) who prided himself on being the fastest wielder of a scalpel in the pre-anesthetic age. Students packed into the gallery around his operating theater, and Liston would wade through the blood of previous operations wearing Wellington boots and challenge his audience to time him. Speed was paramount to Liston, and while he enjoyed breaking records his patients often had much longer-term problems to deal with. One patient had his leg amputated in less than 150 seconds, but such was the good doctor's enthusiasm with the saw that he also removed the poor fellow's testicles. The patient lost a leg, two testicles—and his life, when he died of gangrene soon after.

This was not the full extent of the carnage inflicted by the self-centered surgeon. While performing an amputation on another subject (who also died of gangrene), Liston severed the fingers of his assistant and he, too, died later of gangrene. As the surgeon's scalpel flailed around, it also slashed the coat tails of an onlooker who had a heart attack, thinking the blade had plunged into his vitals. Liston made an indelible impression on all who saw him. He was a large man, six foot two, but moved with a cat-like grace as he leapt upon a new patient, strapped down and prepared for the operation. Liston was a showman and would call to the watching surgeons and pupils, "Time me gentlemen, time me." With a flash of steel he would cut the flesh around the bone—so quick was he that the audience couldn't detect a gap between the sight of flesh being cut and the grating sound of saw on bone. When not using it for cutting, he would place his bloodied knife between his teeth until he was ready to use it again.

There were good reasons for placing such a premium on speed. Before anesthetics, a patient could die from

BELOW **Robert Liston was the celebrity surgeon of his day. He welcomed innovations such as anesthesia.**

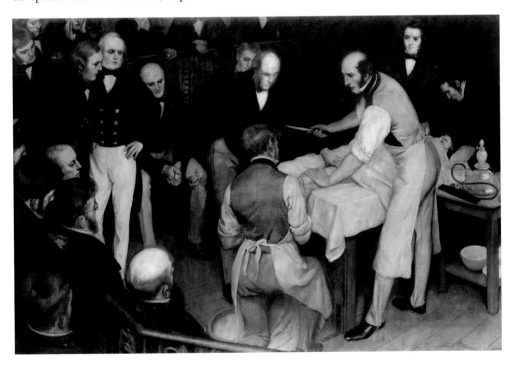

shock brought about by pain or coronary arrest. Surgeons sought to minimize pain by conducting operations as quickly as possible. It seems, though, that Liston also hurried the diagnostic process. A small boy presented with a pulsing tumor on his neck. Another surgeon diagnosed it as a dangerous aneurism on the carotid artery. Liston disagreed, explaining that he had never seen an aneurism on one so young. Acting immediately on his diagnosis, the doctor pulled a scalpel out of his pocket and lanced the offending growth. Not many surgeons slash their patient's throat, but this is what he did in effect, and the poor boy lost consciousness, collapsed, and bled out.

Liston's contributions were not all negative. He did remove a 48-pound (22 kg) tumor from a scrotum in 45 seconds. The patient had brought it into the theater on a wheelbarrow. He performed the first operation in Europe using ether as an anesthetic, and invented several sticking plasters as well as bulldog forceps, still used to lock arteries in modern surgery. In addition he pioneered Liston's flap: a large piece of skin preserved during amputations that is even now used in reconstructive surgery.

The fact that Liston could use knives pulled out of a coat pocket and hold them in his mouth when not using them is a clear indication of an early surgeon's attitude to hygiene and sterilization. Surgeons identified themselves as a superior class of man who were readily identified by their blood- and pus-covered frock coats or aprons. They were equally proud of their surgeons' hands, which gave out an unmistakable waft of dissected corpses, bodily organs, and blood. It was a sign of their professionalism that they could sit down to a hearty dinner and not be bothered by a slight whiff emanating from their fingertips—and, indeed, saw it as a badge of honor.

Making Men Insensible

The practice of surgery changed with the invention of the first effective anesthetic by American dentist William Morton (1819–68). He performed a tooth extraction on Eben Frost on September 30, 1846. This was a momentous occasion as he had knocked the patient out with a handkerchief soaked in ether. Frost miraculously felt no pain and returned to work 20 minutes later.

Morton then built the first anesthetic machine. This was a simple glass globe with one neck allowing fresh air into the globe while another neck was sucked on by the patient. In the globe was a sponge filled with ether. The patient inhaled from one side and was knocked out.

The first full surgical operation was conducted by Professor John C. Warren of Boston on October 16, 1846 on Gilbert Abbot, who had an unsightly but benign arterial tumor on his neck. After 30 minutes' surgery the patient awoke. Although his

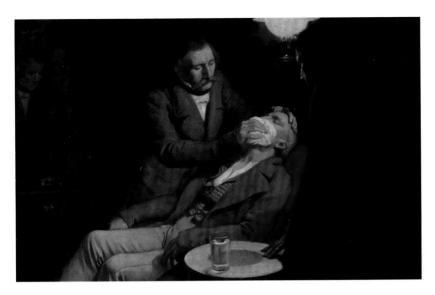

skin had been slashed several times and an artery had pumped out blood before a ligature was applied, Abbot had not felt a thing. History had been made. News of the remarkable discovery soon reached Liston in London. He built a machine just like Morton's and purchased some ether. On December 21, 1846 Liston performed the first British amputation under anesthesia in University College London. Frederick Churchill needed his tibia removed and was knocked out with what Liston called a "yankee dodge . . . for making men insensible." Liston pulled out

ABOVE Eben Frost was the first patient to be knocked out prior to a tooth extraction by his dentist, William Morton, in 1846.

It's All Done, Alice

The first amputation using ether as an anesthetic took place on November 7, 1846, in Massachusetts General Hospital in Boston. Before this, patients undergoing an amputation had to survive excruciating pain. Alice Mohan was a servant girl who had gangrene of the knee joint. The inventor of ether anesthetic, William Morton, knocked out the young girl while Dr. George Hayward performed the procedure. After the operation Alice stirred, woke up, and said to the surgeon that she was ready for him to begin. Hayward reached down, picked up the amputated leg, and proudly showed it to his patient: "It's all done, Alice."

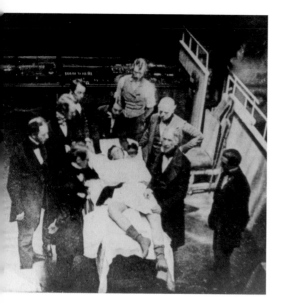

LEFT **A reenactment of the first operation using ether on October 16, 1846. The patient slept through the entire operation, a medical first.**

his favorite knife—it had a notch on its handle for every successful operation—and within 28 seconds the offending limb was removed. The wound was dressed before Churchill awoke. He tried to sit up and said that he had changed his mind and he did not want to have the operation. He, too, was shown the detached limb, but what he said is not recorded.

A new era of modern surgery had begun. No longer would surgeons have to rush to complete an operation. Did Liston slow down? Unlikely.

CHILDBED FEVER AND THE INVENTION OF ANTISEPTICS

Pride and arrogance led to countless numbers of women dying in childbirth or soon after. But the incidence of childbed fever did lead to one positive outcome: the development of sterile medical environments.

For countless centuries and in many countries childbirth was an exclusively female domain. In a European context, experienced midwives would facilitate birth using a blend of inherited wisdom and common sense. "Gossips" often attended and it was their role to ensure that the baby was not swapped at birth with a "foundling," as well as giving moral and physical support. Most births took place in the bedchamber, and though birth was a risky event, mortality rates were generally low. Without formal training, some of the services offered by midwives were less than useful. Concoctions of herbs mixed with alcohol, called a caudle, were provided to facilitate labor. One French publication in 1739 recommended giving the mother-to-be a draft of various ingredients including the opiate derivative laudanum. It also recommended that newborn babies should be washed in beer and butter before having warm wine poured down their throat or squirted up their nostrils. If the child was unhappy, it too should be given a dose of laudanum to settle it down. No doubt the most practical and successful midwives got more work.

Midwives first received official recognition in the early 16th century when a licensing system was established, so that recognized midwives could baptize infants if they seemed destined to die prematurely. They were urged not to use spells, prayers, charms, or witchcraft unless it was approved by the Catholic Church. They were issued with a license once they had taken an oath not to dismember babies, pull off their heads, or swap one child for another. Such things must have happened quite regularly before forceps were available to aid the birthing process.

Nevertheless, into the 19th century, having a baby born at home with an experienced midwife was the safest method of giving birth. Mortality rates among infants were approximately 14 per 1,000, while mothers who died in childbirth were around 2 per 1,000. Once male doctors decided to get involved in the field, the mortality rate soared—all thanks to dirty hands.

Killer of Mothers

Childbed fever, or puerperal fever, is a particularly nasty disease suffered by women who have just given birth. During the Victorian era in Britain (1837–1901) it was the chief cause of mortality among women after childbirth. Approximately 5,000 women died each year during the latter half of the 19th century; this exceeded the deaths from cholera for the

BELOW This Renaissance woodcut shows midwives who appear to be practicing excellent hygiene. This was not always the case: many women died after childbirth.

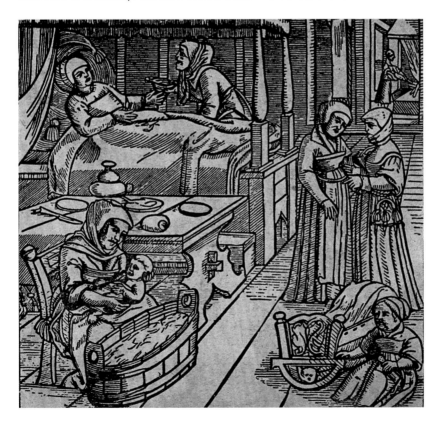

entire United Kingdom. The first known descriptions of the condition date back to at least the 5th century BCE and are found in the writings of Hippocrates. These infections were a very common cause of death around the time of childbirth.

After birth, a woman's genital tract has a large bare surface that is prone to infection. The cavity and wall of her uterus are vulnerable to infection, as is the site where the placenta has been dislodged. Any incidental cuts or abrasions can also invite infection. A range of bacteria can enter her bloodstream through any of these avenues and cause a multiplicity of perilous conditions. The most dangerous microbe is the bacterium *Streptococcus pyogenes*, which is often found in pus-filled carbuncles or pimples. Women who have experienced long and painful deliveries, or lost a lot of blood, are at particular risk of infection.

Once infection had taken hold, the women were guaranteed a painful, prolonged death as pus, blood, and corrupted rotting flesh poured out of their vagina while they were racked by agonizing cramps. Women cried out in agony for days before they died. It would begin between one and ten days after childbirth with a tender uterus that had not returned to its normal size, along with lower abdominal pain. A slight

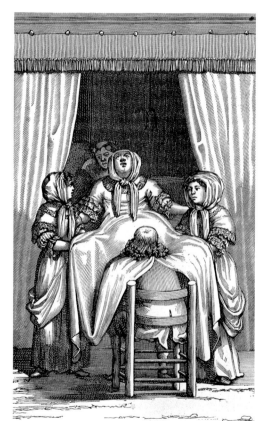

chill was followed by a raging fever above 100.4° Fahrenheit (38° Celsius). Purulent and foul-smelling vaginal discharges featured, and these would be followed by bloody, pus-filled emissions. The patient then became listless before hypothermia, rapid breathing, and the reduction of white blood cells led to a collapse of the immune system. Blood poisoning would then set in before the poor luckless mother died of shock, blood loss, or heart failure.

One would imagine the medical profession would desire to limit the condition, but through a set of misguided policies they actually encouraged it. When a Viennese doctor, Dr. Ignaz Semmelweis, alerted contemporary physicians to a simple cure, he was ridiculed and humiliated to such an extent that he ended his days in a mental asylum.

LEFT **It is to be hoped that this doctor washed his hands before helping the delivery. If not, puerperal fever and a painful death were the likely outcome for the mother.**

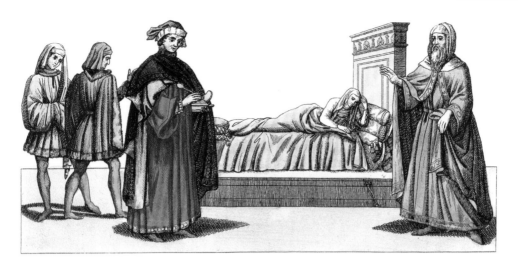

"Doctors are gentlemen and gentlemen's hands are clean." So said the American obstetrician Charles Meigs when the ludicrous idea was put to him that he should clean his hands to cut the incidence of childbed fever in the women under his care. Callous attitudes to women dying in childbirth are not new, and Martin Luther (1483–1546) wrote, "If a woman dies in childbed, that does no harm; that is what they were made for." The male medical profession was usually loath to be involved in obstetrics and many universities refused to teach it, considering the whole field to be ungentlemanly. Oxford and Cambridge teaching hospitals only offered this option to their interns from the 1840s.

ABOVE An uncomplicated delivery was much sought after. Women were advised to write their last will and testament before giving birth.

In an attempt to reduce mortality, maternity establishments or "lying-in" hospitals were instituted throughout Europe. One of the first was in Paris in 1646, and soon many other cities followed suit. Concentrating expectant mothers in purpose-built facilities with neonatal specialists on hand might seem at first sight to be a terrific idea, but in fact mortality rates among young women soared and whole wards were sometimes carried off as puerperal fever swept through the patients. Mary Shelley's mother died in this manner, and maybe her attitude to a callous medical profession epitomized by Victor Frankenstein was a result of this loss. A mortality rate of one in four was common in these wards, and doctors were keen to blame corrupted breast milk or miasma for the infection. Concoctions of herbs, the application of leeches, purging, and bleeding with a lancet were all tried once infection set in, but to no avail.

The hospitals were often run as charitable institutions where women hoped to give birth in a comfortable and safe place and be provided with food, accommodation, and warmth. Male midwives (accoucheurs) delivered the babies and for difficult births a male surgeon would be summoned. In larger lying-in wards 5 to 20 percent died, while in smaller wards severe outbreaks or puerperal fever might see off up to

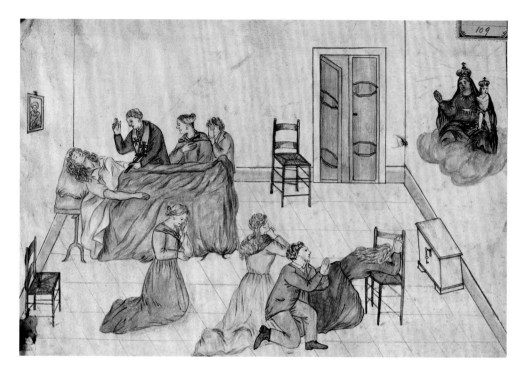

ABOVE **Premature babies had little chance of survival right up until the late 20th century. Here, a family prays for both mother and child.**

100 percent of their patients. Even the most prestigious institution, Queen Charlotte's Maternity Hospital in London, established in 1739, had a mortality rate 17 times higher than women who delivered babies in the worst slums of Whitechapel.

But the doctors and midwives operating in these institutions were themselves the problem. With such a high death rate it was important that surgeons were able to carry out autopsies on deceased patients, so most lying-in hospitals had mortuaries and dissection rooms. Physicians would often dissect dead women to ascertain the cause of death before proceeding to the wards to help with deliveries or physically examine mothers. Gloves were not used, and if instruments were needed they would not be sterilized. Doctors considered it ungentlemanly to wash their hands and were proud of the stink of cadaver on their hands and under their fingernails.

Cleanliness is Key

Some doctors were able to see cause and effect. As early as 1795, Scottish physician Alexander Gordon noted that puerperal fever was seen in women who were attended to by nurses and doctors who had previously attended another sufferer. He believed that he himself had carried the infection to countless women, although he was not sure of the nature of the infection.

In 1843, Dr. Wendell Holmes of Harvard Medical School observed a colleague and a medical student dying of puerperal fever after conducting an autopsy on a woman who had died of the condition. He made the link and suggested that the illness was transmitted on the hands of the practitioner or by the atmosphere that he carried around with him. He noted one case where a doctor removed the pelvic organs of a young woman who died of puerperal fever and put them in his coat pocket before going on to assist a number of women who all died soon afterward. Holmes wrote:

> *In the view of these facts it does appear a singular coincidence that one*
> *man or woman should have ten, twenty, thirty, or seventy cases of this rare*
> *disease following his or her footsteps with the keenness of a beagle, through*
> *the streets and lanes of a crowded city, while the scores that cross the same*
> *paths on the same errands know it only by name.*
> —THE CONTAGIOUSNESS OF PUERPERAL FEVER, DR. WENDELL HOLMES,
> 1909-14

The First Antiseptic

Fresh urine carries no germs, is sterile, and has a long history of use as a wound cleanser. The Spanish Conquistadors (16th century) used it to clean wounds inflicted by the native people's stone weapons. The Romans were aware of urine's antiseptic properties, as shown in the writings of Pliny the Elder (23–79 CE). He described how ground-up burned oyster shells were mixed with old urine—this was used as remedy for running sores and skin rashes on children. Urine was also used to treat corrosive sores, burns, anal trouble, cracked skin, and scorpion bites. Pliny noted that midwives of the time asserted that no better washing medium existed. Urine could be combined with soda to cure head wounds, dandruff, and other spreading sores, particularly of the genitalia. Dog and snake bites were also treated with urine. If pierced with a sea-urchin spine, the sufferer was advised to moisten the spine with a sponge or cloth drenched in urine. Pliny also stated that "every individual benefits most from his own urine."

LOUIS PASTEUR AND JOSEPH LISTER

LOUIS PASTEUR (1822–95) was responsible for several breakthroughs which were then used by Joseph Lister (1827–1912) to improve surgical safety. Pasteur did not invent germ theory but he proved to the medical establishment that bacteria and viruses were respon-sible for many of the ills that beset mankind. He demonstrated that bacteria could sour milk and wine, and invented in 1862 the process of "pasteurization," which involved the boiling and then cooling of liquid to kill bacteria. In 1879 Pasteur discovered his first vaccine and protected chickens from chicken cholera by exposing them to an attenuated form of the disease. He then protected humans by developing vaccines for anthrax, smallpox, and human cholera. In 1885 he performed the first successful vaccination of a nine-year-old boy who had been bitten by a rabid dog.

Joseph Lister was born in Essex, England, and was at the cutting edge of medical practice at the time, attending the first British surgical procedure under

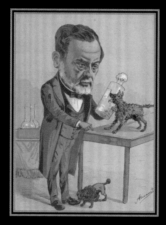

LEFT Among his many achievements, Pasteur invented a vaccination for rabies. However, it must be administered within 24 hours of a dog bite to be effective.

anesthetic in 1846. Reading Pasteur's work on micro-organisms, he used one of the techniques proposed by the Frenchman: covering surgical wounds with dressings soaked in carbolic acid. This vastly reduced the rate of infection. Lister then experi-mented with sterilizing instruments and washing hands, and developed machines that sprayed a solution of carbolic acid onto the patient during surgery. He is now known as the "father of antiseptic surgery."

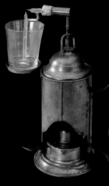

LEFT Joseph Lister used his steam spray to pump a vapor of carbolic acid into operating rooms and hospital wards. This created an antiseptic environment.

Holmes was howled down by his indignant peers, but his treatment was not nearly as bad as that received by Ignaz Semmelweis when he developed his "cadaveric theory." Semmelweis noted that the teaching hospital birthing clinic in Vienna in which he worked had a mortality rate of 10 percent, while a neighboring obstetric clinic in the same hospital had almost no deaths. His clinic performed autopsies on the dead women and they were usually conducted by medical students in his charge. The students and Semmelweis would then attend to patients who were still alive. He noted that the other ward was run by midwives who did not conduct autopsies.

Semmelweis concluded that the death-dealing "cadavers' poisons" were carried into the women's genital organs on the hands of the students and doctors. He took the courageous step of demanding that all on his wards wash their hands in chlorinated lime, and saw an immediate drastic drop in mortality. Hounded out of Austria for his beliefs, Semmelweis ended his days in an asylum, a bitter, humiliated man. It appears that he too died from sepsis infection after an unhygienic procedure. Posthumously his achievements were ranked alongside those of Lister and Pasteur, but it took many years and countless deaths before his ideas were accepted.

In the 1920s, a quarter of a million women died in childbirth in the United States, because America was slow to adopt the basic preventative measures introduced by the likes of Joseph Lister. In addition to his carbolic acid spray, Lister had insisted that instruments, dressings, and surgical gowns be sterilized. These measures were introduced into English maternity hospitals in the 1880s, alongside the use of masks, sterilization of instruments in autoclaves, and the liberal use of disinfectant. Continental and English cases of puerperal fever diminished immediately. Any that did occur were isolated from the general population to limit infection, and antibiotics further reduced infections. Cleanliness was the key and, if only Meigs and his like had not been so stubborn, millions of lives would have been saved.

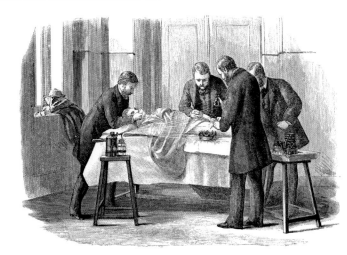

RIGHT **With the spread of Lister's carbolic spray, the mortality rate of those undergoing surgery dropped dramatically.**

5

LEPROSY AND TUBERCULOSIS

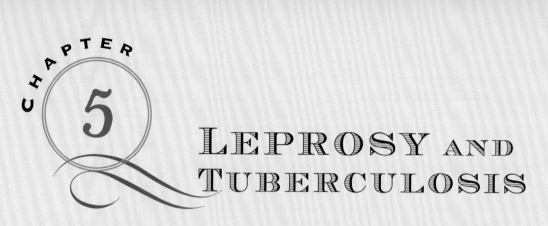

IT MIGHT APPEAR STRANGE TO INCLUDE SUCH DISPARATE DISEASES AS leprosy and tuberculosis, or TB, in one chapter. While tuberculosis ravages the interior of its victim, leprosy is known for the dreadful effect it has on the person's exterior. But both diseases are in fact closely related (caused respectively by *Mycobacterium leprae* and *M. tuberculosis*) and it seems that while one is dominant in a population, the other is submerged. Leprosy was a highly visible illness during medieval times. As tuberculosis gained traction within the European population in the 18th century, leprosy faded into the background, almost as though of its own accord. Leprosy is currently limited to small enclaves where poverty and lack of medical care allow it to survive, but tuberculosis is undergoing something of a renaissance. Antibiotic-resistant strains are making it once again a lethal pathogen infecting millions around the world.

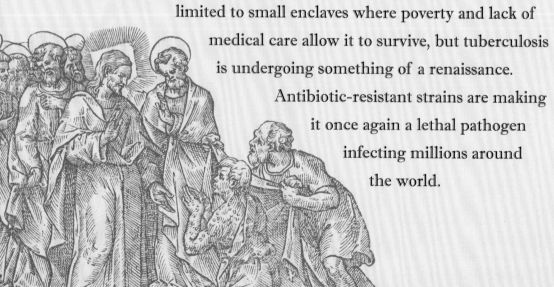

THE STORY OF LEPROSY

Leprosy, also called Hansen's disease, is a chronic infectious disease caused by *M. leprae*, a rod-shaped bacterium, or bacillus. During the period when it is infectious it develops slowly and can take up to 40 years to reveal itself, which makes it difficult to diagnose and aids its spread. It results in horrific skin lesions and deformities on the colder parts of the body such as nose, ears, fingertips, earlobes, and testicles.

Human-to-human transmission is the most common mode of propagation, though chimpanzees, mangabey monkeys, and nine-banded armadillos also carry it. It is believed to be transmitted by nasal discharges, and one-thirtieth of a fluid ounce (1 milliliter—a couple of tiny droplets) of snot carries 1 to 2 million bacteria. It can be contracted through the skin or by spider

Close Cousins

Leprosy and tuberculosis may seem very different but the germs that cause them, *Mycobacterium leprae* and *M. tuberculosis*, are close cousins. They are members of a family of slender, rod-shaped mycobacteria that evolved in the sea hundreds of millions of years ago before adapting to live in fish, reptiles, birds, and mammals. Both bacilli are likely to have moved into human populations about 10,000 years ago and may have leaped the species divide from mice or water buffaloes. Though it is impossible to know exactly when the two cousins first infected humans, what is clear is that infection with one bacillus will create resistance to the other.

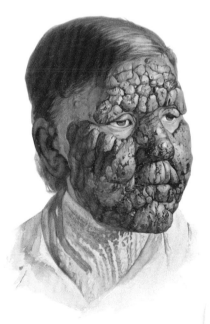

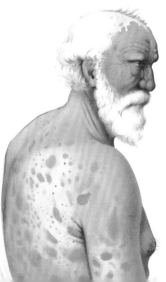

LEFT Leprosy leads to thick disfiguring tissue building up on the extremities before spreading to other parts of the body.

RIGHT Leprosy destroys nerve endings. This means that sufferers are less aware if they suffer wounds or infections, leading to further complications.

bites, but this is rare. Placental and mammalian milk transfer can occur, ensuring that it stays in the family.

Numbness, and loss of ability to detect heat or cold in extremities such as fingertips, progresses until all sensations of pain, touch, or pressure are lost. Painless ulcers and flat, pale areas of skin follow, before larger ulcerations lead to facial disfigurement and loss of digits. Lesions occur particularly on the hands, face, and knees. Children and grown males are twice as likely to contract leprosy as adult women.

Leprosy leads to a range of deformities. The most common form results in nose and eyebrows being eaten away. Deformities arise in the hands and feet due to motor nerve damage. "Anesthetic deformities" arise when wounds are not attended to due to lack of nerves (and therefore absence of pain) in the digits. Wounds can suppurate, bruise, become scabby, and bleed without the patient noticing. Eyes become desensitized, leading to a collapse in the blink reflex. The patient stares continually while detritus builds up on the eye, resulting in eye infections and eventually blindness.

An Outcast's Disease

Leprosy was one of the most feared diseases in history—not because it was easily communicable, but because of the horrific appearance sufferers presented to the world. As the infection ate away digits, limbs, and facial features, many lepers stank of rotting flesh and gangrene. Cleaning became a big issue as pieces of skin or flesh could come away with clothes or drop off in the street.

The illness had no cure, so many ancient societies sought to isolate or stigmatize sufferers. Holes were inserted into church windows so that lepers could see a church service but not join the rest of the congregation. Special clothes would be worn, and in many communities bells were issued to lepers so that they could warn people to stay away or to prepare alms.

The first written record appears in an Egyptian papyrus dated to around 1550 BCE. It was present in the Indian subcontinent well before this; a recent fossil find from Rajasthan, India, has been dated to around 4000 BCE. The disease is mentioned in an ancient Hindu text, the *Atharva Veda*, written before the first millennium BCE. In 758 CE, it is believed that Empress Komyo set up the first leprosy hospital in Japan.

The Japanese sense of aesthetics produced a particular horror of leprosy. Sufferers were disowned by their families, and had any resources or assets stripped from them. Neighbors denounced them and would shun them until they left to be confined in purpose-built shrines, where they died as miserable beggars. They were not allowed to receive education or run businesses. Often a family would secretly take their offspring to a leprosarium so as not to be disgraced within their community.

During the early and middle medieval period leprosy became one of the worst scourges in society. One of the first leprosy hospitals was established near Canterbury, England, in 1085, and by 1350 there were at least 300 "lazar houses" (leper hospitals) in the British Isles alone. It had been present in England as early as 400 CE, where skeletal remains display the characteristic ravages and deformities produced by the disease.

BELOW On the Indian subcontinent lepers were condemned to live as beggars among stray dogs, shunned as "outcasts" below even the "untouchables."

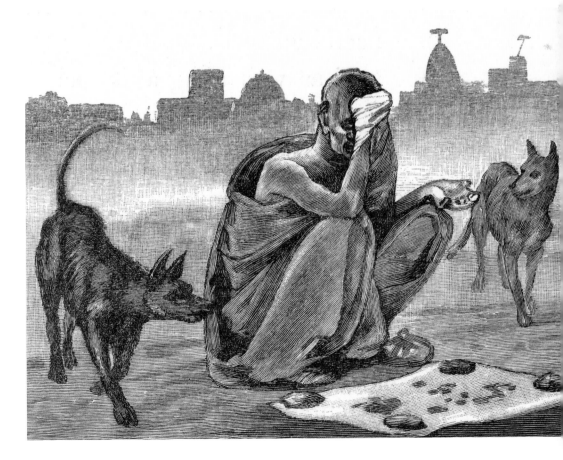

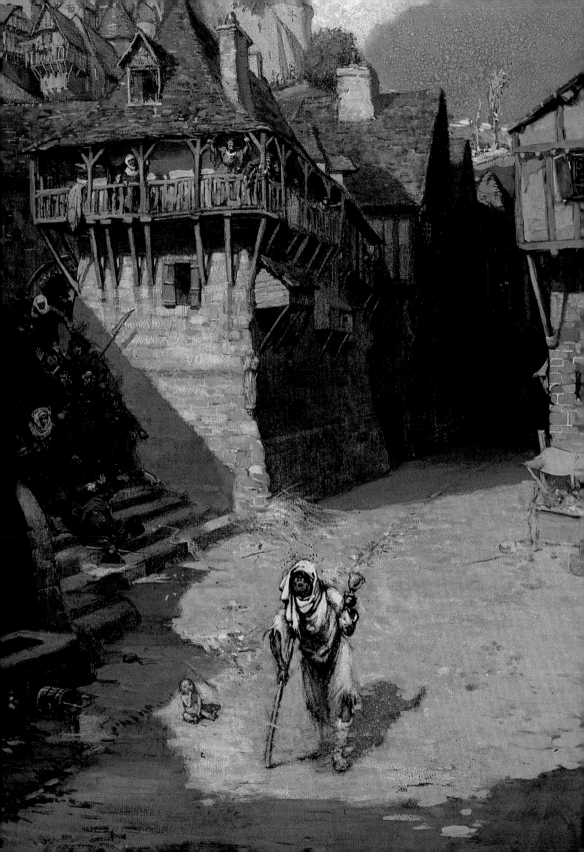

TREATMENT AND PREVENTION

There were undoubtedly wide variations in the ways in which lepers were identified and treated in medieval Europe. The archetypal perception involves lepers as outsiders and outcasts carrying a bell or clapper to warn people of their disgusting presence, or confined in horrific conditions in leper hospitals until they died a miserable death. Evidence now available seems to contradict this: In fact, most skeletons that have signs of leprosy were buried in community graveyards, indicating that they lived within the community rather than being shunned.

It would also appear that the care offered in leper hospitals (called lazar houses after the patron saint of lepers, St. Lazarus) was of a high order, and churches, nobles, and towns were willing to make the unfortunates' lives as easy as possible. Christians must have reflected that Jesus was sympathetic to their plight and cured several lepers, according to the Bible, with the command "Be clean." Cures and preventatives ranged from prayers to the adoption of a healthy diet, herbal baths, bloodletting, and ointments. By 1400 the worst of the scourge was over and leper hospitals were either closed down throughout Europe or converted into hostels for the aged or pox-ridden.

LEFT Leprosy sufferers were required to wear distinctive clothing to cover the horrific appearance of their gangrenous limbs.

BELOW By law, lepers in medieval Europe had to ring a bell or sound a clapper to alert other people to their approach.

Leprosy Today

Today there are several effective treatments for leprosy, including the drugs promin and dapsone, both developed in the 1940s. The use of these drugs slashed the number of lepers in the 20th century. Nevertheless, approximately 250,000 cases are detected every year, concentrated in Africa, Asia, and Latin America. Multi-drug therapy that combines dapsone, clofazimine, and rifampicin reduces the effects of the disease, but it is in no way eliminated despite 95 percent of the world's population being immune.

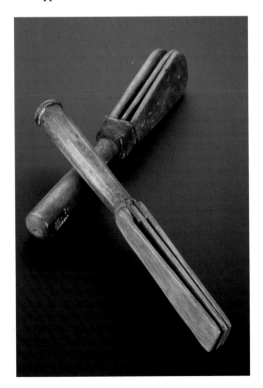

THE RISE OF THE WHITE DEATH

With leprosy on the wane by the early 15th century, tuberculosis became a greater threat. As urban populations grew, the transmission of tuberculosis became easier due to overcrowding; this seems to have reduced the incidence of leprosy.

Tuberculosis has been known by many names throughout history, names that hint at the dreadful toll it takes on human life. The Greek term *phthisis*, which can be interpreted as meaning "consumption," showed how even in a healthy Mediterranean climate it infected people and "consumed" them seemingly from within. Other names included "the white death," "the great white plague," "the robber of youth," "captain of death," "the graveyard cough," and the "king's evil."

Tuberculosis is a wasting disease that infects the lungs, leading to consumption, where victims cough out their life force as the dreadful *Mycobacterium tuberculosis* eats away at the lung until a final coughing fit expels what remains of the lung tissue, which by this fatal stage looks like a bloody bunch of grapes.

Tuberculosis is one of the most ancient scourges and was present in many animal populations before the most primitive primates evolved. It is a great survivor among illnesses and it should be no surprise that it is making a comeback against the puny defenses we have been able to mount against it.

BELOW **The crowded tenements of industrial age Europe were the perfect breeding grounds for tuberculosis.**

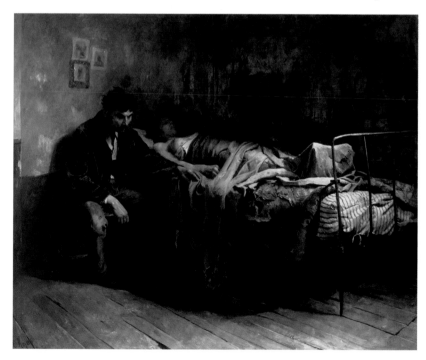

Mycobacterium tuberculosis in its slow-burning epidemics may have killed more people than any other disease, and it is likely that its ancestors were around as long ago as 150 million years. Its current distribution in its many forms equates with the distribution of landmasses during the Jurassic period when most landmasses were united in the supercontinent Gondwanaland.

Current methods of genome sequencing place an early strain of *M. tuberculosis* in East Africa as early as 3 million years ago, where it must have been present in early hominid populations as they evolved in the rift valleys. *Mycobacterium tuberculosis* is such an efficient predator that it does not have to morph to adapt to new environments—hence its low mutation rate. This allows fairly accurate tracking of the evolution of its genome, and it seems that 35,000 years ago the variants *M. africanum*, *M. canettii*, and *M. bovis* evolved from a common African ancestor. Fifteen thousand years ago in East Africa one of these strains evolved into the six modern forms (clades) that are present today. These clades have further evolved into modern strains that are still evolving. It can be presumed that earlier strains were taken out of Africa as *Homo erectus* colonized many of the world's landmasses and that these strains were replaced just as *H. sapiens* replaced their ancient hominid ancestors.

ABOVE This small sample of sputum is teeming with *Mycobacterium tuberculosis*. A single sneeze could spread up to 40,000 infectious droplets.

EARLY REPORTS OF TUBERCULOSIS

The earliest unambiguous detection of *M. tuberculosis* involves evidence of the disease in the remains of bison in Wyoming dated to around 17,000 years ago. It is likely that the current strains infecting humans originated in bovines and then transferred to the human population due to domestication. Both strains of the tuberculosis bacterium share a common ancestor, which could have infected humans as early as the Neolithic revolution.

Paleopathological evidence dates back to 8000 BCE and signs of spinal tuberculosis have been found dating from the Neolithic era in 5800 BCE. The earliest record of tuberculosis in complete corpses is found in ancient Egyptian mummies where the characteristic spinal deformities of Pott's disease have been found. These characteristic humps that form as the spinal column decays were also depicted in Egyptian art, demonstrating the presence of spinal infections. *Mycobacterium tuberculosis* DNA has also been sourced from mummified lung tissue, proving the presence of the pulmonary variety. Early biblical texts such as Deuteronomy and Leviticus mention the disease under the name *schachepheth*. Mesopotamian tablets from the 7th century BCE may allude to this disease; one inscription reads: "What he coughs up is thick and frequently bloody. His breathing sounds like a flute. His hand is cold, his feet are warm. He sweats easily, and his heart activity is disturbed."

Indian texts describe tuberculosis as early as 1300 BCE and Chinese sources do the same in 2700 BCE. A "wasting disease" was described in one of the earliest medical works, the Chinese *Huang Ti Nei-Ching* of the third millennium BCE. Evidence of bony tuberculosis is abundant in Peruvian mummies, proving that it was established in the indigenous populations of the Americas well before European invasions.

Bronze Age and early Iron Age Greeks were aware of the disease, and Homer's epic poem the *Odyssey,* transcribed in the 7th or 8th century BCE, refers to "grievous consumption which took the soul from the body" and caused a person to "lie in sickness . . . a long time wasting away." Classical Greeks named the disease *phthisis* (which can mean "consumption" but can also be interpreted as "dwindling" or "wasting away") and Hippocrates was able to specify its symptoms as well as the age range of its most likely victims: between 18 and 35. He considered pulmonary phthisis a hereditary disease, as it so commonly occurred throughout a whole family.

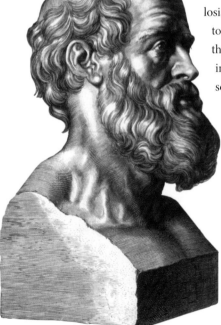

During the Middle Ages, the impact of tuberculosis seems to have lessened. This may have been due to the decline of urbanization with the collapse of the Roman Empire, but it also resulted from the increased incidence of leprosy which entered something of a "golden age" of physical deformity and horror. Nevertheless, it is suspected that some powerful individuals such as St. Francis of Assisi died from tuberculosis.

LEFT **Hippocrates wrote one of the earliest descriptions of tuberculosis. He thought it was hereditary, as whole families were often struck by the disease.**

An Urban Plague

By the 1800s tuberculosis began to sweep through Western nations in an epidemic tsunami. A new virulent strain may have evolved that led to horrific death rates in Northern Europe and North America of above 1 percent of the population per annum. This was exacerbated by the poor conditions experienced by those living during the Industrial Revolution in crowded tenements with little or no sanitation. Particularly in the winter months when little fresh air was allowed, young and old developed the wrenching cough typical of the disease.

London provides a good example of how newly industrialized cities allowed the spread of tuberculosis among the urban poor. The crowded slum tenements facilitated the transmission of the disease—called in England "the white plague"—through sneezing, coughing, and spitting. The cramped dwelling conditions of these slums were perfect for the rapid transmission of bacteria. Added to this were the leaking privies and pervasive dampness which allowed the bacteria to survive away from their human hosts for a bit longer, ensuring more people were exposed and infected.

BELOW **Tuberculosis was one of the chief causes of death in industrial England. Enclosure saw millions of people forced from the land into crowded unsanitary slums.**

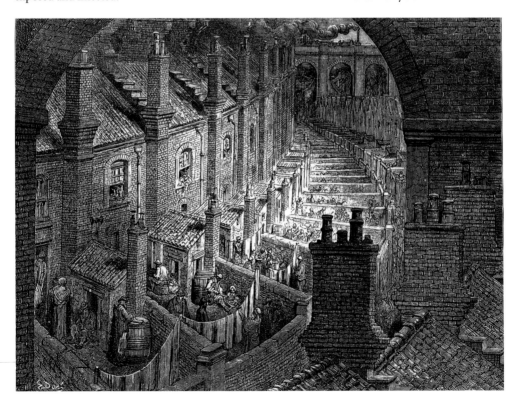

PULMONARY TUBERCULOSIS

Ninety percent of tuberculosis infections are pulmonary (within the lung). It can take fewer than eight or ten bacteria to cause an infection and each droplet of sputum exhaled in a cough or sneeze usually contains two to three bacilli. This makes tuberculosis one of the more easily communicable diseases.

The bacteria make their way deep into the lungs where they are ingested by macrophages. Macrophages are the first line in the body's defensive system and act as guards to keep the unwanted organism out of the lower respiratory tract. If the defense is successful the tuberculosis bacteria will be entrapped within several layers of calcified tissue, causing harmless tubercles. These can remain dormant for the remainder of the host's life, causing no illness or symptoms. This form is known as "latent tuberculosis." Patients with this form will give a positive result if tested and can develop the full-blown disease later in life if their immune system becomes weaker.

BELOW Wealthy sufferers of tuberculosis retired to sanatoriums in the hope that fresh air would cure their affliction. This was usually in vain, and death was their constant companion.

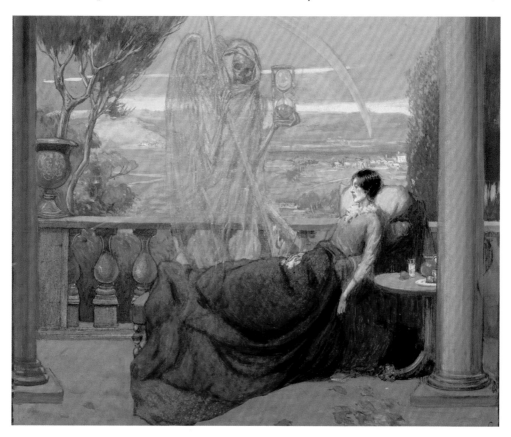

Wasting Away

From the 1700s through to the 1890s, folklore often associated tuberculosis with vampires. When one member of a family died from it, the other infected members would lose their health slowly. People believed the original person caused this, with tuberculosis draining the life from the other family members. TB was also prevalent in the upper classes, leading to a fashion where looking pale and wasted was desirable. This is echoed in today's "Gothic" look. Authors such as Dostoyevsky, the Brontës, Dickens, and Byron described how generations of youth were destroyed physically, while their spirits remained bright. Famous men and women over the ages suffered from this disease. Notable among them were the poets John Keats and Percy Bysshe Shelley, the authors Robert Louis Stevenson, Emily Brontë, and Edgar Allen Poe, and the composers Niccolò Paganini and Frédéric Chopin, to name but a few. Tuberculosis was seen in the same light as the drugs and alcohol that have killed the brightest and best in modern media such as Jimi Hendrix and James Dean.

Edgar Allan Poe described his young wife, Virginia, who had tuberculosis, as being "delicately, morbidly angelic." In 1842, while they were having dinner, Virginia had a sudden coughing fit and hemoptysis and Poe remarked: "Suddenly she stopped, clutched her throat and a wave of crimson blood ran down her breast . . . It rendered her even more ethereal."

Emily Brontë described the tuberculous heroine in *Wuthering Heights* as "rather thin, but young and fresh complexioned and her eyes sparkled like diamonds." Emily, her four sisters, and her brother Branwell all died in childhood or young adulthood from tuberculosis, and their mother also died of the disease.

BELOW Frédéric Chopin was one of the many artistic geniuses to contract tuberculosis. He died in 1849, despite receiving the best medical care available at the time.

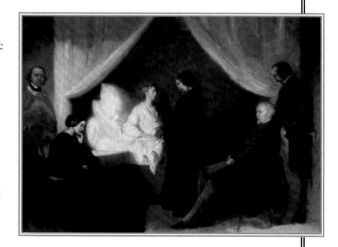

But in many individuals this is only the opening skirmish and, while these macrophages can kill and consume the deadly bacteria, the invaders have millions of years of accumulated evolutionary attack strategies to ensure their survival. *Mycobacterium tuberculosis* (the most common species in humans) often continues to live and replicate within the macrophages that continue to attack the invaders, but as the *M. tuberculosis* can't be killed giant multinucleated cells are created within the lung.

If the invading strain is too virulent or the host's defenses are too weak, this giant cell bursts and bacteria flood into the lungs and throughout the body, most commonly into the lymph nodes. The body is aware of the infection and after four weeks marshals more phagocytic cells that enclose the new infections; these form new growths $^1/_8$ inch (3 mm) in diameter, called miliary tuberculosis because the nodules resemble the grain millet.

After this, the infection develops into its deadliest form. Within the lungs, these cells of infection join and reproduce to form larger granuloma (a collection of immune cells gathered together to form a small lump of inflamed tissue) where the mycobacteria interact with the cells of the immune system and suppress them. Necrotic (dead) cells within these granulomas cause the body to create pus and fluids that fill the surrounding tissue. It is during this phase that patients will begin wasting away due to continual coughing as they seek to expel poisonous fluids from the lungs.

Doctors performing autopsies on TB victims describe how the lungs are so filled with chunks of dead bacteria-ridden flesh that they have the texture of soft, crumbly cheese. These cheese-like suppurating sores within the lungs are called "caseous necrosis" (cheese-like dead flesh). However, these necroses are not the only way in which the immune system tries to protect the lungs. Often the necroses are replaced by scar tissue called "fibrosis." This fibrosis does not contain lung alveoli, which are essential for conveying oxygen from the airways to the bloodstream, and this contributes to reduced lung function in the patient. As the patient coughs up cells and fluids from

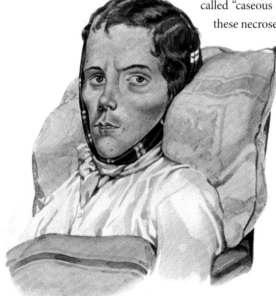

LEFT **A patient suffering from pulmonary tuberculosis, with characteristic swelling of the lymph nodes around the neck.**

these decaying pieces of lung they not only transmit millions of bacteria into the atmosphere but cause the holes in the lungs to grow until large cystic cavities called "empyema" develop. As the lung tissue dissolves, a foul stench is emitted from the corroding soft tissue, breathing becomes more difficult, and the patient wastes away, eventually dying of heart failure and lack of oxygen.

In some tertiary cases of infection, just before the patient dies they cough up large chunks of lung that look like bunches of grapes. These consist only of connective tissue and major air vessels, as the rest of the sponge-like material has been consumed by the bacteria.

SPINAL TUBERCULOSIS

Also known as Pott's disease, spinal tuberculosis is a particularly nasty form of TB that results from the bacteria leaving the pulmonary system and invading the spinal column. Instead of large chunks of lung being eaten away by the bacteria, the cartilaginous joints between the vertebrae are attacked. This usually occurs either on the upper or lower spine, the first leading to a characteristic hump.

The intervertebral disk space is attacked, and if two or more disks are attacked in this manner they cannot receive nutrients and begin to collapse as they die. This crumbling spinal matter then interferes with nerves within the spine, leading to paraplegia (paralysis of the lower body).

Symptoms include agonizing back pain, fever, night sweats, a hunched posture that minimizes spinal articulation, anorexia, protruding spinal mass, and muscle weakness. Eventually the entire spine can collapse, leading to paralysis and death. Abscesses often form and drain pus into the surrounding soft tissue, causing pain distant from the actual sight of infection. Hips and knees can be attacked in this manner. Children are the most susceptible to Pott's disease, which accounts for about 2 percent of tuberculosis cases.

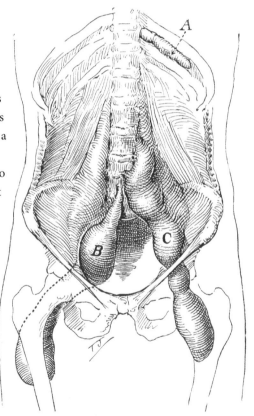

ABOVE **Vertebral tuberculosis causes the formation of large abscesses and eats away at the connective tissue of the spine.**

115

EXTRA-PULMONARY TUBERCULOSIS

Tuberculosis can be spread through the vascular system, lodging in other parts of the body. The lining of the abdominal cavity is attacked, leading to swelling, tenderness, and appendicitis-like pain. The bladder can be infected, making for extremely painful urination with blood in the urine. Bones may be eaten away, leading to pain similar to the symptoms of chronic arthritis. TB that infects the tissues covering the brain is known as tuberculous meningitis. Symptoms include fever, a constant headache, neck stiffness, nausea, and drowsiness that can lead to coma. Tuberculosis may also infect the brain itself, forming a mass called a "tuberculoma." This may cause symptoms such as headaches, seizures, or muscle weakness. Reproductive organs can be attacked, leading to large painful lumps in the male groin and infertility in women. The kidneys are susceptible and develop scarring and swelling that leads to an eventual breakdown in kidney function. More serious is when the pericardium (the membrane around the heart) is infected, leading to fever, enlarged neck veins, shortness of breath, and heart failure, as the organ becomes surrounded by inflamed tissue.

BELOW The use of breathing apparatus (as pictured here) may have led to some short-term relief; however, it could not stop the decomposition of lung tissue.

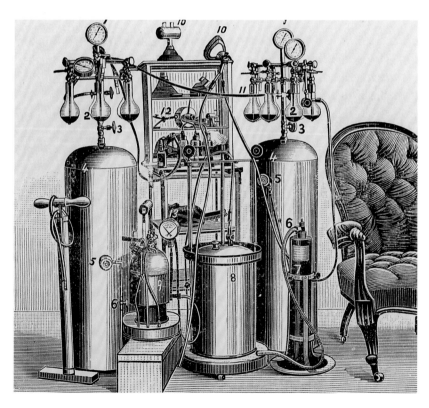

SCROFULA

One of the most distressing illnesses in recorded history would have to be scrofula. This is also caused by the tuberculosis bacteria. The lymph nodes around the neck become infected and enormously swollen. In a new tuberculosis infection, the bacteria may travel from the lungs to the lymph nodes that drain the lungs. If the body's natural defenses can control the infection, it goes no farther, and the bacteria become dormant. However, very young children have weaker defenses, and in them these lymph nodes may become large enough to compress the bronchial tubes, causing a brassy cough and possibly a collapsed lung. Occasionally, bacteria spread up the lymph vessels to the lymph nodes in the neck. An infection in these may break through the skin and discharge pus. Otherwise, they cause huge growths under the chin and around the neck, causing distress to all who suffer from the illness and all who can see its effects.

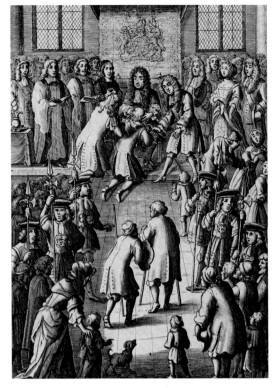

ABOVE **King Charles II of England performing the "king's cure" on a scrofula sufferer.**

Historically this was cured by "the king's cure": Monarchs would touch the disfiguring ailment or give a gold token that the victim wore around the neck. The Frankish King Clovis (ca. 466–ca. 511 CE) was the first recorded monarch to treat with the "royal touch" those who were suffering from this disfiguring complaint. Robert the Pious, Edward the Confessor, and Philip I of France all dedicated many resources to trying to cure the disease. Charles II of England touched 92,102 infected subjects during his 25-year reign (1660–85).

THE LYMPH NODES AROUND THE NECK BECOME INFECTED AND ENORMOUSLY SWOLLEN. IN A NEW TUBERCULOSIS INFECTION, THE BACTERIA MAY TRAVEL FROM THE LUNGS TO THE LYMPH NODES THAT DRAIN THE LUNGS.

CURE AND PREVENTION OF TUBERCULOSIS

To cure tuberculosis the Romans recommended bathing in human urine, devouring wolf liver, and drinking elephant blood. Early Arab scholars advocated consuming ground crab shells mixed with asses' blood.

In Hippocrates's era (4th century BCE) patients were nursed in temples and treated with plentiful and good food, milk (particularly asses' milk, as it was thought that asses were not prone to phthisis), and exercise.

The Roman emperor Marcus Aurelius's physician Galen recommended fresh air, milk, and sea voyages for its treatment. This Greek physician described phthisis with fever, sweating, and coughing of blood-stained sputum, and found tubercles in phthitic lungs that he called *phûma*. He considered it to be infectious and warned against close contact with sufferers. Pedanius Dioscorides, a Greek army surgeon in the service of Nero (54–68 CE) and author of *De Materia Medica*, recommended "warming drugs" such as animal fats; and Tertullian (160–225 CE) prescribed butter boiled with honey.

BELOW **Desperate patients would try anything. Many tonics contained amphetamines, alcohol, and morphine, a "guaranteed pick-me-up."**

In 1840, just as industrialization took off in England, there were 68,000 recorded deaths from tuberculosis. Some of these deaths may have been attributable to cross-infection from non-pasteurized milk.

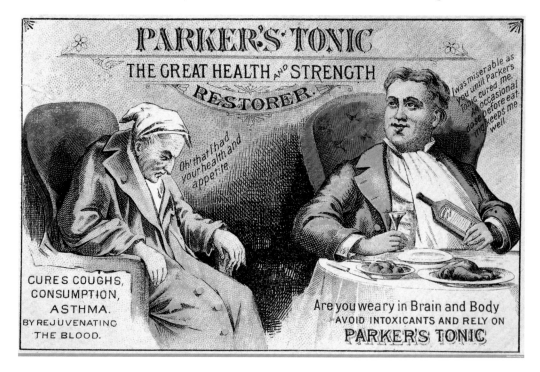

PARKER'S TONIC
THE GREAT HEALTH AND STRENGTH RESTORER.

Oh! that I had your health and appetite.

I was miserable as you until Parkers Tonic cured me. An occasional dose before eating keeps me well.

CURES COUGHS, CONSUMPTION, ASTHMA. BY REJUVENATING THE BLOOD.

Are you weary in Brain and Body AVOID INTOXICANTS AND RELY ON PARKER'S TONIC

English authorities began some of the earliest public health campaigns and encouraged families to boil their milk; this brought a noticeable drop in deaths from this infection.

In Europe, incidence of tuberculosis increased in the early 1600s and peaked in the 1800s, when it was responsible for 25 percent of all deaths. Thanks to new treatments, by the 1950s mortality had decreased by nearly 90 percent. Innovations in public health reduced the rates of tuberculosis even before the use of antibiotics.

In 1946, the antibiotic streptomycin was developed, making effective treatment and cure of tuberculosis possible. Prior to the introduction of this drug, one difficult treatment used (other than sanatoriums) was surgical intervention. This included the "pneumothorax technique," during which an infected lung was collapsed in order to "rest" it and thereby giving the tuberculous lesions time to heal.

In 1953 there were 84,000 cases recorded in the United States, but by 1984 the figure was reduced to 22,000. This led to a tragic miscalculation by the medical establishment. Research dropped to almost nil and interns were not trained to look for the warning signs and symptoms. Equipment such as isolation wards, ultraviolet lights, and ventilation systems were discarded or neglected. By 1985 cases again began to increase.

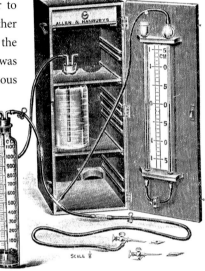

BELOW Pneumothorax apparatus such as this were used to collapse the lungs of tuberculosis patients. It was thought that the collapsed lung would heal more readily before being reinflated.

TUBERCULOSIS TODAY

Tuberculosis has returned with a vengeance. Since the *Mycobacterium tuberculosis* bacterium can live within macrophages for years and lie dormant until a carrier's immune system is weakened, tuberculosis was able to form an unholy alliance with the new disease AIDS. This was combined with the collapsing American health system, which did not cater for the needs of poorer members of society. The disease began to thrive among drug addicts, prostitutes, the homeless, and prisoners. Many of these marginalized individuals were refused care or did not seek medical help. Many patients who were fortunate enough to receive medication began to feel better after two weeks and this caused them to quit the treatment before the microbes had been dealt with. The suppressed bacteria were able to come back with a vengeance and develop resistance to antibiotics. In the 1980s many strains could resist one type of antibiotic but now they can resist five or six. A new generation of superbug has been unwittingly created. The new strains reap a doleful harvest from the homeless crowding in shelters, subways, and bus stops. In addition, the prevalence of recirculation systems in planes and buildings is causing the disease to infect what were previously considered low-risk populations.

A new generation of Typhoid Marys (see page 198) is moving through both developed and developing countries. After dropping out of treatment they relapse and present again. A new type of antibiotic is administered, as they no longer respond to the original medication. As soon as symptoms abate, they clear out again. Difficult to trace in countries with poor social security networks, the carriers disappear into their usual haunts, spreading new potent strains among their luckless peers. Many are hospitalized up to five or six times, leading to multiple infections and new strains in one carrier.

The subsequent resurgence of tuberculosis resulted in the declaration of a global health emergency by the WHO (World Health Organization) in 1993. Tuberculosis rose by 30 percent in Europe, while in AIDS-stricken Africa it rose by 300 percent in the 1990s. Asia also saw huge increases, and the disease is still a major public health

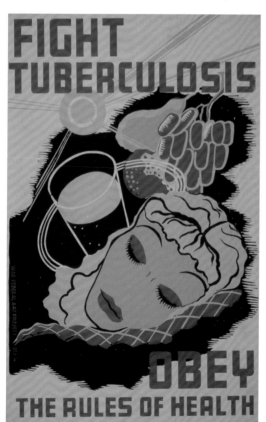

problem today. In 2011, 8.7 million people were infected with tuberculosis with between 1.4 and 3 million deaths occurring every year. This amounts to 9,000 deaths every day, far exceeding the numbers killed by malaria or cholera. New surgical procedures are being developed to remove infected lung tissue, but while some of these newfangled techniques may be appropriate in a Western economy, the misuse of antibiotics has led to what is essentially a new plague with a new pathogen that has been able to use its millions of years of evolutionary biology to present a "clear and present danger" to humanity.

LEFT **Fresh air, a healthy diet, and a good night's sleep were advertised as preventatives for tuberculosis in this 1936 poster. Only penicillin would give an effective cure.**

RENÉ THÉOPHILE HYACINTHE LAENNEC

R ENÉ LAENNEC (1781–1826) WAS a French physician credited with inventing the stethoscope. In 1816, he was determined to check on the lung function of a well-endowed young woman he suspected might have been infected with tuberculosis, but he was uncomfortable with the idea of pressing his ear against her ample chest. He had an inspirational thought: He rolled up his notebook and, applying one end to her chest, he listened through the other end. He was astounded to hear a clear heartbeat ringing out like a clarion bell, as well as her breath passing through her lungs.

Soon after this Laennec constructed a hollow wooden tube and named it the stethoscope, from the Greek *stethos* (chest) and *skopein* (to look at). It evolved into its modern form in the early 1850s.

A brilliant anatomist, Laennec was able to use his stethoscope to chart the course of pulmonary tuberculosis and developed a terminology that reflected how it ate away at the lungs with abscesses, ulcers, and finally the pus-filled cavities called empyema where the lung tissue is entirely eaten away.

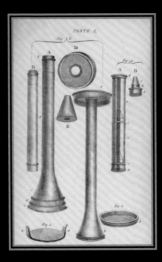

The first phase was the "miliary" or "millet seed" phase of phthisis. The lungs seek to isolate the bacteria, forming hard nodules of scar material that eat into lung tissue. These then develop into the "caseous" or "cheese-like" phase. This would have been better described as "Swiss cheeselike" cavities as the lung tissue begins to break down, forming cavities and empyema. Finally, the tubercles grow to such a size that they fill with pus and make breathing all but impossible.

Laennec developed other terms to describe the doctor's practice and the sounds that emanated from his patients' lungs. He was the originator of the terms "ausculta-tion" (listening carefully), "rhonchus" (a whistling or snoring sound), "pectoriloquy" (the chest speaks), "egophony" (resonance), and "râle" (a rattling sound), of which there were five types including "crépitant" (crackling). Laennec's intimate under-standing of tuberculosis came at a cost: He died of the disease in 1826.

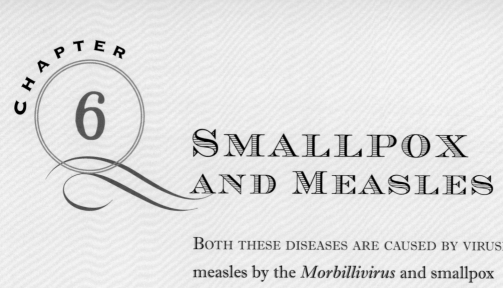

6

SMALLPOX AND MEASLES

BOTH THESE DISEASES ARE CAUSED BY VIRUSES: measles by the *Morbillivirus* and smallpox by the *Variola* virus. They are *exanthemata*: diseases that cause rashes and eruptions characterized by pustules. They often follow hard on each other's heels and are difficult to separate. In the 10th century CE a Persian physician made a distinction between the two diseases, but presumed they were two phases of the same disease. Both are crowd diseases that do not require an animal carrier; they rely on a carrying human population.

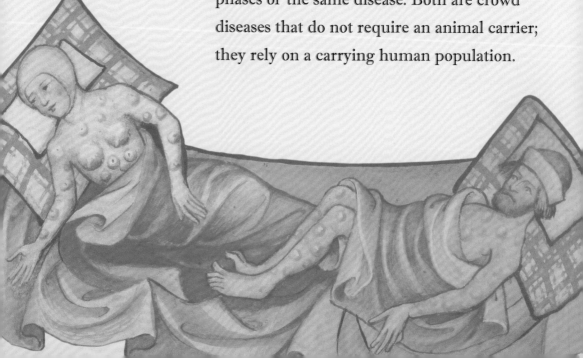

SMALLPOX

Variola is a grenade-shaped virus with nodules covering its surface. Having evolved for millions of years, it has relatives throughout the animal kingdom. Cowpox, horse pox, crocodile pox, insect pox (which acts by liquefying the insect's interior), and chicken pox are examples of these. Its rich heritage is evident in its genetic makeup which contains 187 genes; this is in contrast to the AIDS virus which only has 10. It is an airborne virus which initially sets up shop at the back of the throat, allowing transmission through saliva or coughing. A sneeze or a cough from an infected person sends thousands of virus-laden particles into the air. Transmission can also occur if a person comes into contact with the pustules. Clothing, blankets, or other materials that have been on the body of a smallpox victim carry the disease and if anybody uses them they can also catch it. Dead bodies covered with pustules are highly contagious, and breezes can blow the virus around.

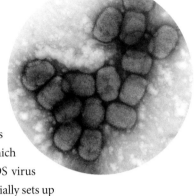

ABOVE **A colorized transmission electron micrograph of the deadly smallpox virus.**

BELOW **Having one's skin covered in smallpox pustules was painful enough, but they often also coated the tongue, mouth, and throat.**

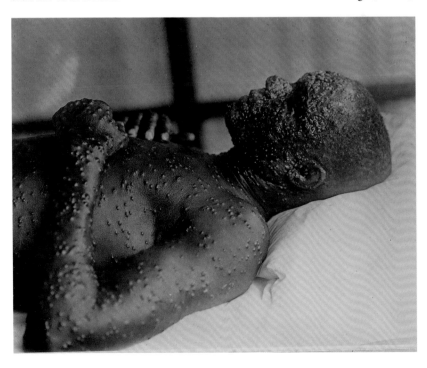

Smallpox moves from the respiratory system before passing to the lymph nodes to invade its host's cells, where it replicates. The virus then indicates to the host cell that it wants to exit; the host cell is programmed to bond with another cell, allowing the virus to move into the new host and continuing the process. This intracellular contact allows replication to occur without alerting the body's antibodies to react. This initial incubation period usually lasts 10 to 12 days.

Once sufficient viruses have developed, they rupture the host cells and enter the bloodstream before migrating to the spleen and bone marrow. Initial symptoms are similar to other viral infections, with fever, muscle pain, malaise, headache, nausea, and vomiting. This "pre-eruptive" stage lasts two to four days.

Patients then move into the most dangerous stage of the infection. A rash covers much of the body, which is followed by small spots that grow into pus-filled pustules called "variolae," from the Latin term for spotted. These also appear on the mucous membranes of the mouth, tongue, palate, and throat. Any swallowing or eating action ruptures these hypersensitive pustules, leading to the throat being covered with infectious pus and fluid which is rapidly transmitted into the air. This means of propagation has two horrific effects on humans. Young

BELOW This graphic Japanese illustration of smallpox traces the development of the pustules from their closed, benign state to their infectious stage, when they became weeping, open sores.

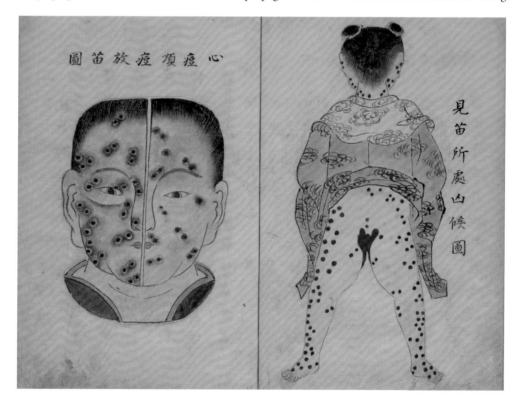

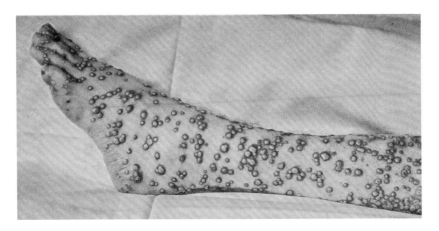

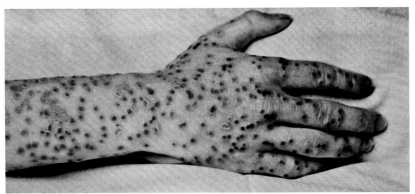

and old find it too painful to drink, leading to death through dehydration; and the disease's highly contagious nature means each person who is infected goes on to spread the disease to an average of four other people. Transmission can also occur if people come into contact with the pustules, which after several days dry up, crack, and become scabs before shedding. Even shed pustules are highly infectious, and only when totally healed do people stop being carriers. People who die before shedding the pustules can remain contagious for up to a year if buried in a warm, dark location.

ABOVE **Three stages of variolous lesions are shown. The pus-filled pustules (as shown on the leg) dry out and form scabs. On the hand the scabs are drying out while on the forearm the scabs are being shed.**

The variolae break out between 24 and 36 hours, after which no new ones develop. The pustules itch and burn so fiercely that sufferers often feel as if they are on fire. When the pustules finally burst on around the tenth day, the victim is covered in oozing sores that smell like rotting flesh.

TYPES OF SMALLPOX

Smallpox was initially simply called "pox" until it was given its new title to distinguish it from the "great pox," otherwise known as syphilis. It was subdivided into *Variola minor* which was relatively benign and only killed 1 percent of those who were infected, and *V. major* which had a mortality rate of 30 to 35 percent, and was most likely to leave unsightly pockmarking, blindness from ulcers on the cornea and, in some cases, arthritis.

The pox is further subdivided into four other classifications: ordinary, malignant, hemorrhagic, and modified. Malignant and hemorrhagic are the most lethal.

Ordinary Smallpox

Ordinary smallpox was still a nasty disease. Ninety percent of sufferers had this type. The first symptoms were small macules—colored lesions under the skin's surface. By the second day of the rash, the macules began to protrude above the skin and became papules—lesions up to ½ inch (13 mm) wide, filled with pus. On the third or fourth day the papules became pustules, filled with an opalescent fluid which then turned

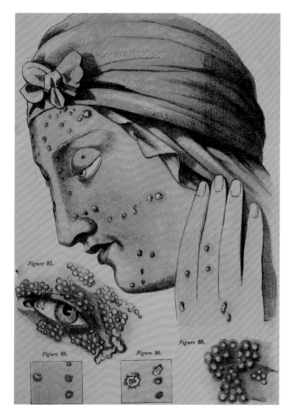

Figure 87.

Figure 89.   *Figure 90.*   *Figure 88.*

cloudy over the course of the next 24–48 hours. The pustules were densest on the face and the extremities, including palms and soles. The contents of the pustules was not actually pus, however, but rather tissue debris. It would take up to the sixth or seventh day for all of the skin lesions on the body to take this form, then, between the seventh and tenth day, the pustules grew to their maximum size. By this stage they were typically raised, round, and firm to the touch—almost like a small bead in the skin. They were embedded very deeply in the dermis (the inner layer of the skin). Over the course of the following week fluid would gradually leak from the pustules.

LEFT **This illustration shows different types of variolae associated with smallpox, chicken pox, and cowpox.**

By around day 14 the pustules would deflate and begin to dry up and form scabs. Sometimes the scabs would merge together—this was known as aconfluent rash. It would adhere to clothes or bedding, resulting in large sections of skin peeling off when the patient moved.

Malignant Smallpox

Malignant smallpox was also known as flat smallpox, as the lesions remained almost level with the skin. Children were the main sufferers of this disease, which killed almost 90 percent of victims. The children were struck with severe flu-like symptoms before the virus materialized in soft and velvety vesicles concentrated in the mouth and on the tongue. This was often followed by blood poisoning and death.

Hemorrhagic Smallpox

The hemorrhagic strain of smallpox was also known as the "black pox," as the pustules formed and burst under the skin, making it look charred and black but still smooth to the touch. One of the first symptoms was bleeding in the eyes, turning the whites of the eyes a dark red. While the skin turned black and the eyes turned red, the virus would attack the internal membranes of the body. Those lining the eyes, lungs, liver, kidneys, heart, and intestines were all attacked, leading to excessive internal bleeding. The ovaries, bladder, and testes were often attacked and the sufferer's entire body collapsed from the inside, leading to excruciating pain and suffering. Death occurred after approximately eight days of infection. Two percent of smallpox cases resulted from this form of the disease and it was almost invariably fatal.

Modified Smallpox

Modified smallpox was the most benign form of the virus and could be confused with chicken pox. It was rarely fatal and struck when a previous inoculation had worn off. The initial inoc-ulation usually granted about 30 years' protection.

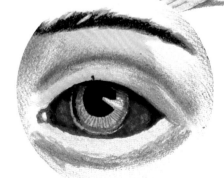

RIGHT This patient suffered from hemorrhagic smallpox. One of the first symptoms was the eye turning red, heralding widespread internal bleeding, which was almost invariably fatal.

PLAGUE OF THE AGES

It is likely that prehistoric hunter-gatherer peoples may have on occasion been infected with the original smallpox virus from rodents; however, it was only during the Neolithic Revolution that smallpox became a permanent feature of human existence, and the virus developed means to target human cells. Once the virus was able to move from person to person there was no need for it to mutate to a more benign form, as there were always enough new hosts. It established itself in the Fertile Crescent of ancient Mesopotamia (modern-day Iraq and Iran) by 8000 BCE, and as early as 3000 BCE Egyptian documents appear to refer to a smallpox-like disease—though these and later references could equally refer to measles outbreaks. Egyptian traders probably spread the illness to India by 1500 BCE, and the Hittite Empire was struck in 1350 BCE. The mummified body of Ramses V, the Egyptian pharaoh who died in 1157 BCE, shows clear signs of pockmarks on his face and hands. Thucydides, the Greek historian, described the outbreak of an epidemic in Athens in 430 BCE, in which citizens who appeared to be perfectly healthy suddenly developed a raging head fever followed by red inflammation of the eyes. Their breath became "unnatural and unpleasant" due to the bleeding from their throat and tongue. The skin also turned a livid red and small pustules and ulcers broke out. These began on the head but soon spread over the whole body. Very few survived the ordeal, and, Thucydides noted, "even when people escaped its worst effects, it still left its traces on them." This plague of smallpox contributed to the Spartan victory over Athens, one of the many times crowd diseases have altered history.

ABOVE **Ramses V was one of the last great pharaohs. He survived an early bout of smallpox, and the pockmarks are visible on his mummified corpse.**

It is possible that the Roman plagues of 165–180 CE and 251–266 CE were caused by these two pathogens, *Morbillivirus* and *Variola*. Both cause rashes and eruptions. In 164 CE soldiers dispatched to Syria to put down a revolt brought back with them what seems to have been smallpox. It raged for 14 years, killing one-third of Italy's population and 7 million throughout the empire. Periodic visitations over the next centuries fatally weakened the Western Roman Empire. The symptoms included violent vomiting, diarrhea, fever, skin lesions, and a sore throat. It was transmitted by skin-to-skin or skin-to-clothing contact. It is likely that the Huns first picked up the virus during the 4th and 5th centuries CE in their travels north of India before carrying it to China, where it was called Hun pox or Mediterranean pox.

Disease of the Gods

Such was the terror felt toward smallpox that some cultures invented deities whom they would try to placate in order to avoid their wrath. Shitala, the Hindu goddess of smallpox, appeared in India about 3,000 years ago. Her name meant "the cool one" and if she possessed you, cool drinks were required to get her to leave.

BELOW **The Hindu goddess of smallpox and her frightening attendants were given offerings to keep them away.**

The Chinese had T'ou-Shen Niang Niang, who particularly targeted beautiful children so that she could ravage their fair countenances. She roamed for victims at night, and parents would cover their children's faces with grotesque images drawn on paper. Christians prayed to St. Nicasius of Reims; not only had he survived the disease in his youth, but legend has it that he also carried his head to the church steps after Germanic heathens beheaded him.

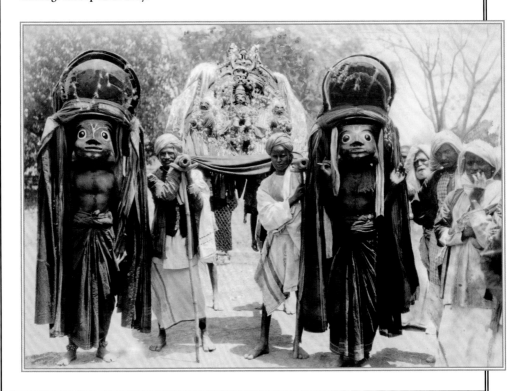

ALL THANKS TO A COW

A cow called Blossom and a milkmaid called Sarah can be credited with indirectly saving millions of lives. Edward Jenner (1749–1823) was a doctor in the dairy region of Gloucestershire, England. He made the keen observation that milkmaids who caught cowpox from infected udders were not struck down by smallpox even though it infected those around them. Pondering the situation, he decided to see if this observation had a practical outcome. In May 1796 a local milkmaid, Sarah Nelmes, became infected with cowpox, probably caught from Blossom. This disease is similar to smallpox and produces pustules on the skin, but it is not lethal. Jenner lanced one of Sarah's pustules and scratched it into the skin of his gardener's son, James Phipps. Six weeks later he did the same thing but with fluids taken from a smallpox victim. Young James remained healthy. Jenner carried out the same procedures on his own son and he too was not infected. The first vaccinations had been performed, although they were not called this until Louis Pasteur (1822–95) named the procedure, deriving the term from the Latin word for cow: *vacca*.

BELOW Edward Jenner's techniques, though parodied in this cartoon, were copied by physicians throughout Europe. Millions were saved, all thanks to a cow called Blossom.

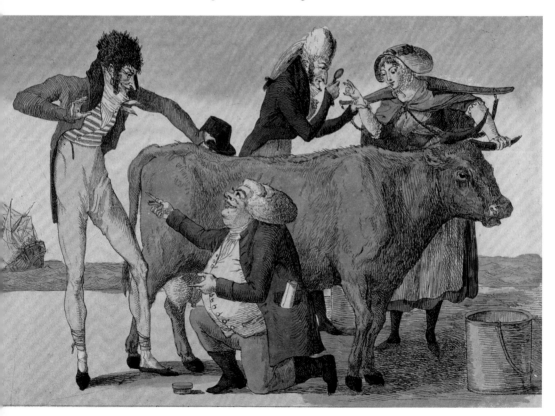

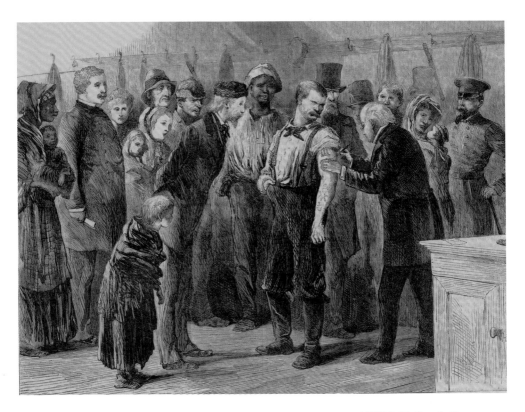

BATTLING THE POX

Inroads were made into smallpox from the 1800s when widespread inoculations were performed. A worldwide program to finally eradicate the disease was carried out in the 1970s and now it exists only in two biohazard labs. Not many diseases can be entirely written of in the past tense. Smallpox can, though, because it currently resides only in two vials at opposite ends of the earth. The last cases of smallpox in the world occurred in an outbreak of two cases in 1977, after which the WHO (World Health Organization) declared that the pestilence had been eradicated. This led to the decision to destroy all known stocks of the disease except for vials in the United States and Russia. In 1986 WHO recommended destroying these last examples too, but both countries refused to destroy their stocks in the interests of future research.

ABOVE Initially only the wealthy could afford to be inoculated. However, in 1863 mass production of the smallpox vaccine was developed. Here, New Yorkers are given protection in 1872.

MEASLES

In Western countries today, measles is seen as an almost harmless disease that causes a bit of a skin rash and fever. Worldwide, however, it is the fifth highest cause of death in children, and the fatal complications can include pneumonia and encephalitis (inflammation of the brain.)

The symptoms initially are a low fever, general niggling discomfort, a dry cough combined with a runny nose. Red and bluish spots appear inside the mouth and the rash begins on a child's hairline before spreading to the rest of the body, causing extreme discomfort. If an individual's defenses are overwhelmed, diarrhea and vomiting can lead to dehydration and death.

A Force to Be Reckoned With

By the Middle Ages measles and smallpox had entrenched themselves in European populations, mainly attacking the young, who then developed some resistance provided they survived. By the 17th century it seems that smallpox developed again into a lethal strain, killing 40 percent of those it infected even in the Old World. Queen Elizabeth I of England nearly died, and thereafter filled her pockmarks with a cosmetic largely made up of distilled baby fat. Mary II of England, Peter II of Russia, and Louis XV of France all succumbed, and, as if in a cosmic revenge for the deaths in the New World, young Louis I of Spain was killed by smallpox in 1724. By the latter half of the 18th century it is estimated that 400,000 Europeans died of it each year.

Measles too continued its deadly work. It killed 30 percent of Fijians when it reached those islands in the 1870s and did the same in Samoa, Hawaii, and West Africa. Eighty percent of Maoris in New Zealand fell to these two diseases. Smallpox is estimated to have killed 400 million people in the first half of the 20th century before it was eradicated.

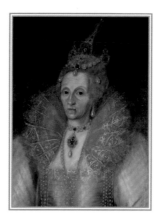

ABOVE **Queen Elizabeth I is said to have filled her pockmarks with a combination of chalk and baby fat.**

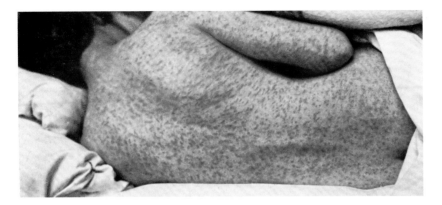

The measles virus is higly infectious. Small samples of virus from an infected person's cough or mucus can survive on dry surfaces for up to five hours. The tiniest amount can then be transferred into a new host's mouth if they eat without washing their hands. Airborne particles are similarly contagious. It is estimated that nine in every ten people who have not been immunized, or have no resistance, that come in to contact with an infected person will develop the symptoms, which usually appear 10 to 12 days after infection. It was this virulence that made measles such a killer in indigenous populations in the New World.

ABOVE Back of a female patient showing a case of measles. The measles was less deadly to Europeans than smallpox. Nevertheless, it was very unpleasant.

It is likely that measles evolved in animal hosts and crossed the species divide in Sumer around 3000 BCE; diseases such as bovine rinderpest and canine distemper are possible origins.

NEW WORLD SCYTHE

Mexico's population before its conquest by Europeans is estimated to have been approximately 20 million. After 100 years it had dropped to 1 million. But it wasn't Spanish gunpowder, steel, crossbow bolts, or lances that killed the native population; it was a combination of European diseases, especially smallpox and measles, which decimated these once proud peoples.

The key to European domination of the mighty Aztec and Inca empires stretched back for millennia. The domestication of fowl and cattle had given Europeans a higher resistance to several diseases, including smallpox. Smallpox is related to *Vaccinia* virus in cows, *Ectromelia* virus in mice, and pox infections in fowl and pigs. Measles is related to a virus that causes distemper in dogs, rinderpest in cattle, and swine fever in pigs. The indigenous inhabitants of Mesoamerica and North America had no tolerance to such viruses and millions of people perished.

Why the native population had no tolerance to these Old World viruses is still something of a mystery. It appears that their ancestors only left the Old World behind approximately 12,000 years ago, when many European diseases must have been developed or developing. It is possible that the epic migration through the icebound strait of Beringia may have acted as a cold filter killing many existing microbes, and the trek no doubt killed any carriers weakened by disease.

The Spanish conqueror Hernán Cortés landed on the coast of Mexico with 600 Spaniards in March 1519. Montezuma II believed Cortés was the god Quetzalcoatl, so he and his party weren't immediately captured and sacrificed to one of the many bloodthirsty Aztec deities. They were initially feted as divine ancestors, but were eventually chased out of Tenochtitlán (now Mexico City) with their tails between their legs, losing around two-thirds of their force. The reinvigorated Aztec warriors under the dynamic new emperor Cuitláhuac routed the Spanish and seized many prisoners, carrying them up to the great pyramid in the sacred precinct for sacrifice.

Cortés was nothing if not determined and he returned repeatedly to renew the battle. He had reinforcements from the Spanish colony of Hispaniola and they brought with them the smallpox virus, which had decimated the native population of those islands several years earlier. A Marxist interpretation would argue that one man can't change history, but one man did fatally weaken the *Mexica*, as the Aztecs referred to themselves.

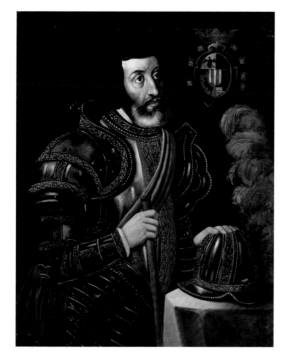

An African slave, Francisco de Eguía, accompanied the Spanish and for two weeks he was expelling germs before the disease finally carried him off. Not a "minor" smallpox strain, but definitely a virulent major strain, it was horrendously lethal. It was a "confluent infection," in which the pustules attack the skin so violently that they all coalesce together to form large suppurating sores covering much of the body. Individuals were covered from head to toe and so awful were the pustules that whole slabs of skin would come off when

LEFT **Cortés did not only bring Christianity and modern weaponry to the New World: He also brought smallpox.**

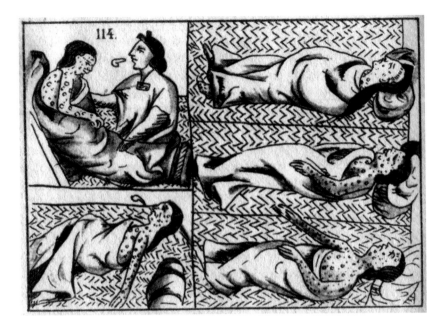

the infected sufferers moved. For 60 days the disease raged in the capital and may have killed upwards of 120,000 people. Many survivors were pockmarked or blinded.

The Spanish Franciscan Toribio de Benavente Motolinía (1482–1568) wrote a vivid description of the impact the new disease had on the indigenous peoples. Since they had no remedy, more than half of them died. Motolinía described how they "died in heaps, like bedbugs." He noted that, since the entire population fell sick at once, none could harvest or prepare foods, so many died of starvation. Often, a whole family would be wiped out. The locals and the Spaniards could not cope with the number of corpses, and so it was common for houses to be pulled down over dead families, so that the ruined house became their tomb.

Throughout Central America, the Mexica and their vassals fled from the scourge. They fled on foot or by boat along rivers and on to the coast. This resulted in the real tragedy. Smallpox incubates for 10 to 14 days, so an apparently healthy refugee could be welcomed by family or friends hundreds of miles from where he had set out, before he broke out in the contagious pustules. It reached Mayan lands, where the disease was called *nokakil*—the great fire—as it ran unchecked through their population.

Combining with his Tlaxcalan allies, Cortés once again besieged Tenochtitlán, building a small navy, and fighting house-by-house and street-by-street. The Mexica were initially victorious but one thing fatally weakened them: Smallpox killed at

ABOVE The Aztecs were hit by a strain of smallpox so virulent that the pustules amalgamated to form sores covering the whole body. As they sat up from their mats, their skin would peel away.

least 25 percent of the population and much of the warrior class. The Spaniards said that they could not walk through the streets without stepping on the bodies of smallpox victims. Cortés wrote "A man could not set his foot down, unless on the corpse of an Indian."

The story of the Mexica was repeated throughout many of the peoples of the New World. The effects of smallpox and other diseases such as measles, influenza, typhus, and diphtheria were devastating. The Inca probably could have held off Francisco Pizarro's forces if their numbers hadn't been decimated by repeated outbreaks of smallpox. One infected European was all it took to kill countless numbers of natives.

OLD WORLD VIRUSES CAUSE CARNAGE

The devastation caused by imported infectious viruses occurred throughout Continental America and thousands of tribal groupings that have left no historical record perished. The Cherokee population fell by 75 percent during an outbreak in 1674. Successive outbreaks in 1729, 1738, and 1753 killed those without an immune response from previous outbreaks. In the 1770s, 30 percent of Amerindians died on the northwest coast of America, and in the 1830s the previously untouched population of Inuit in Alaska lost at least 50 percent of their population.

In British Columbia and Washington State the "great smallpox" epidemic of 1862 began in an encampment of Amerindians. The government ordered them to return to their homes, resulting in a rapid spread of the disease that killed approximately 75 percent of the tribespeople. In 1868 the Mapuche, indigenous inhabitants of Chile, almost died out after the Chilean military purposely infected them. Even the nomadic plains tribes such as the Sioux could not escape smallpox's wrath, although only an estimated 15 percent died.

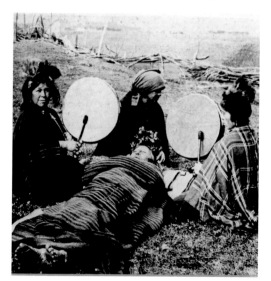

LEFT **Prayer and magic were the only treatment the indigenous peoples of North America had access to. Populations such as these Mapuche in Chile began to recover only in the 20th century.**

The northeastern tribes of North America were hardest hit for several reasons. The five nations of the Iroquois confederacy lived in densely populated encampments with large intergenerational lodges and relied on agriculture for most of their food-stuffs. They also enjoyed extensive trade routes with neighboring peoples, such as the Susquehannock and Onondaga nations. This dense population started to suffer as soon as Europeans visited the area in 1609. They did have resistance to quite a few illnesses endemic to the region, such as dysentery, viral influenza, pneumonia, viral fevers, American trypanosomiasis, roundworms, and syphilis, but had no immunity to the host of Old World diseases, such as smallpox, typhus, measles, diphtheria, influenza, scarlet fever, chicken pox, and tropical malaria.

Once infection hit an indigenous community, any response they took seemed to make things worse. The crowded lodges lacked facilities to dispose of waste. The inhabitants traditionally visited sick relatives and cared for them, therefore exposing themselves to infection transmitted by weeping smallpox pustules. The elderly and young were particularly hard hit as they were most likely to die from infection. This led to a breakdown in normal cultural practices, which served to worsen the epidemic. Often the survivors would run away and let the sick die. The living were unable to bury the dead. They were left for vermin to prey upon. These panicked reactions led to further deaths. Abandoning food sources led to weakness within those not infected, allowing pathogens easier access to a weakened immune system. Many sufferers who might have recovered would die when abandoned, and their rotting flesh hosted bacteria eating the decaying flesh as well as a host of other viral infections. Those people fleeing spread pathogens to uninfected populations.

Another commonly observed response was suicide. Many people deprived of kith and kin, knowing what would happen if captured by a hostile tribe and racked with grief, chose to kill themselves rather than face an uncertain future. Whether a society was matrilineal, as the Iroquois, or patriarchal, the death of lawmakers and leaders made it more difficult for a tribe to rebuild and resist outside aggression.

Measles continued to follow on the heels of smallpox carried by troops, mission-aries, colonists, fleeing natives, and sailors. By 1529 two-thirds of the surviving indigenous peoples were wiped out. Honduras, Mexico, and the Incas were attacked two years later. In Peru repeated infections reduced the Inca population from 8 million to 1 million between 1553 and 1791.

Over four centuries the indigenous New World population fell from perhaps 100 million to 10 million. The study of ice cores reveals that greenhouse emissions dropped noticeably in the 16th century due to this carnage. Only in the last hundred years did the indigenous populations throughout the Americas begin to grow as persecution ceased, immunity grew, and diseases were eradicated or controlled.

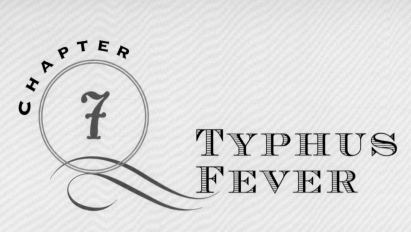

TYPHUS FEVER

MUSKET BALLS, BAYONETS, SABERS, SWORDS, ROUND SHOT, shrapnel, and shellfire were all able to reap a deadly harvest in the revolutionary wars from 1792 to 1815. But it was not this lethal array of weapons that brought down Napoleon's empire—it was typhus. A minuscule bacterium called *Rickettsia prowazekii*, carried in one of the meanest of creatures, the louse, decimated European populations from the 16th century right up to the end of World War I.

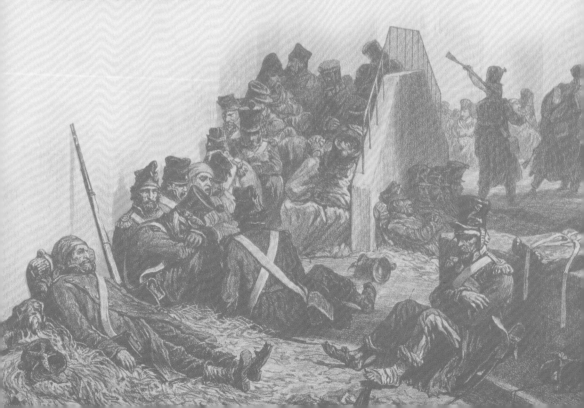

THE SPOTTED FEVER

Typhus was first used as term in the 18th century. It is derived from the Greek word *typhos* that translates as "hazy" or "foggy." This reflects one of the earlier symptoms of the disease, which is characterized by dullness or even stupor. Other early names were "spotted fever," commonly used in England, "red cloak" (*tabardillo*) in Spanish, or "the rash" (*Fleckfieber*) in German.

The *Rickettsia prowazekii* bacterium is transmitted by *Pediculus humanus corporis*, the common body louse. Adding to the dangerous nature of the disease is its comparatively long gestation period. Ten or twelve days after being bitten, a patient might experience a slight chill accompanied by a vague sense of confusion. This soon passes and the victim will most likely discount it as a momentary aberration. But this is just a temporary lull as the bacteria colonize the body before the onset of a full-blown bacterial assault. During this time the *Rickettsia* will have invaded host cells and churned out millions of copies of its DNA. The cells most at risk are those that line the veins and capillaries throughout the entire body. The infected cells swell and leak their deadly cargo into the adjoining tissues, killing the flesh and producing necrotic cells. A victim begins to rot from the inside.

A dull headache can often burst forth into a blinding migraine that entirely incapacitates the victim. This is due to the leaking blood vessels causing encephalitis, which results in swelling in the brain and its lining. This can be accompanied by joint pain, confusion, coughs, low blood pressure, and severe muscle soreness. A livid red rash resembling fleabites can break out and cover the whole body except for the face, the palms of the hands, and the soles of the feet. It is this unique feature that allows the disease to spread so virulently.

During Napoleonic times, if an infected soldier could still march, his uniform would cover the rash and he would stay with his unit, thereby spreading the disease. These spots, too, were a symptom displaying the breakdown of the vascular system as blood clots formed in even the tiniest of veins. Bright light caused agony to sufferers and many described how

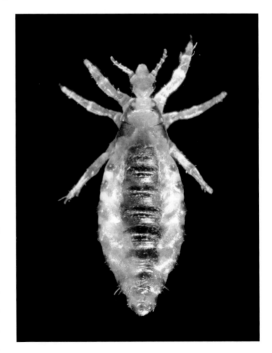

ABOVE **The body louse is found in all human populations around the world. When it carries the typhus bacterium, it becomes a lethal killer.**

sunlight felt like daggers penetrating to the back of the brain. Another characteristic was the disgusting odor emitted by those infected, further reinforcing the idea that the illness was caused by miasma. This was all accompanied by a fever reaching 104° Fahrenheit (40° Celsius), which would cause the lice to evacuate their host in search of a milder climate.

As the disease entered its final phase after eight or so days, victims would begin rambling deliriously, conducting discussions with friends and family far away. Sometimes they would throw off their clothes and race about like a mad person, gabbling furiously. As the blood vessels became constricted with dead cells, oxygen was unable to reach the extremities, leading to gangrene, which commonly occurred on fingers, genitals, and nose as the victim rotted away, leaving a foul stench.

Rickettsial pneumonia occurred when the blood vessels in the lungs gave up and the lungs' alveoli filled with blood, preventing oxygen entering the bloodstream. Unconscious patients lost their gag reflex, allowing infected saliva to flow into the lungs, further inhibiting the uptake of oxygen. Organs such as the kidney would fail due to lack of oxygen. The ravaged vascular system meant that many died of blood loss, not because the patient was bleeding externally, but because the sieve-like veins allowed plasma to leak into the surrounding tissue. Cardiac arrest often killed the victim as the heart tried to pump blood through innumerable clots and perforations in the veins, but found the job too difficult and simply shut down. Many fell into a depressed stupor and died quietly as the disease ravaged their innards.

When autopsies were performed on cadavers, little red blood remained in the bodies. Rather the organs appeared to have been soaking in a saline-like solution and only the lungs were filled, like a sponge, with black, clotted blood.

TINY PASSENGERS

Pediculus humanus corporis is the common clothing louse, or human body louse, which has many nicknames such as "cootie" or "grayback." It is related to other lice which live on humans, and probably became a distinct species several hundred thousand years ago when early humans started wearing furs and hides. As the hair of early humans receded, our ancestral louse had to specialize in order to survive the harsher, less hairy, environment. One type evolved modified claws to allow it to grip the fine, dense hairs on the head; this common head louse does not carry typhus. The second type evolved into "crabs," a flat, nasty little critter with its legs sticking out horizontally from its body so that it can hang on to widely separated pubic hairs or eyelashes. The third type is the body louse, which should really be

RIGHT The dreadful conditions on the Eastern Front in World War I saw a resurgence of typhus. This 1919 poster shows a louse shaking hands with death.

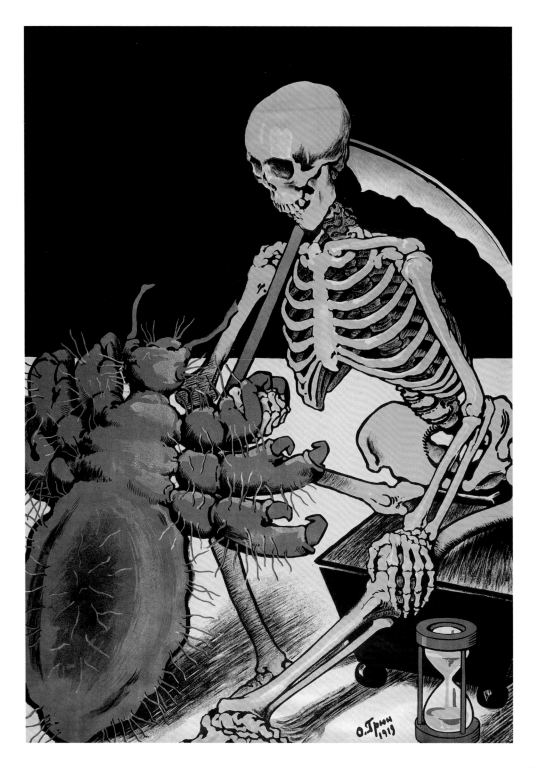

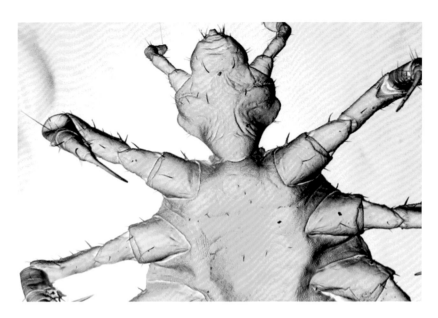

ABOVE **Body lice spread wherever there is poor hygiene, particularly in jails, armies, and among the poor. Their claws allow them to hold on to clothing, making them hard to eradicate.**

called the clothes louse as that is where it lives when not feeding, and where it lays its eggs. Such is the cunning of the body louse that it camouflages itself to suit its host. Lice in Africa are black, the North American type is brown to match the indigenous population, and the European louse is gray-white. These creatures are all distinct from lice that live on our closest genetic ancestors—gorillas and chimpanzees. Genetic studies indicate that these lice became divergent species about 4 million years ago, which would indicate that that is the approximate date when we separated genetically from our cousins. Lice that live on humans are unable to feed on other animals and will die rather than drink the blood of any mammal except for their natural hosts.

The louse is most commonly found in areas where clothing comes closely into contact with the body, for example, the waistline, neck, groin, and armpits. They also hide in seams and linings, making them hard to eradicate manually, and clothes require steaming or chemical treatment to eliminate any infestations. Nits (louse eggs) are laid at about 20 a day for a month and cemented onto body hairs and clothing fibers. If not controlled, lice can multiply into plague proportions; there are many accounts where liberated inmates of concentration camps were asked to strip off and their entire skin seemed to crawl as thousands of lice sought to avoid sunlight.

Lice thrived in the early Christian era and the medieval period, when it was considered sinful to be too clean. This and the growing urban concentrations of the Renaissance allowed lice to entrench themselves in European societies.

THE PERFECT CARRIER

Ectoparasites (parasites that live on the surface of the skin) cause much discomfort, leaving painful bites that need to be scratched. It is only when they carry endoparasites, such as the deadly *Rickettsia prowazekii*, that they become dangerous.

After hatching, the young lice immediately begin to feed during the night and day, particularly when their host is quiet. They molt three times before reaching sexual maturity and after 21 days they can begin reproducing. Adult lice can live for another 30 days and feed often, engorging themselves on their host's blood. They discharge large pellets of dark red excrement, and the chief means by which people are infected by *R. prowazekii* is when they scratch the feces into sores or cuts, allowing the bacteria to enter the bloodstream.

The louse is also killed by the *Rickettsia* bacteria. When lice feed upon an infected person, they also become infected. The organisms enter the louse's intestinal tract where they multiply furiously before being passed in the louse's waste. Infected lice die within ten days.

When lice are present in huge numbers there are other ways that they can infect humans. If scratched by their host, pieces of the lice may be rubbed into any slight tear in the skin. If lice feces are allowed to dry, they become a fine powder which becomes airborne, allowing the feces to be inhaled into the human respiratory tract. It appears that bacteria can live in lice feces for several years, leading to recurrent pulses of infection if discarded items of infested clothing are worn again.

BELOW **This disinfection crew in German East Africa was part of government's countermeasures to the 1902 typhus epidemic.**

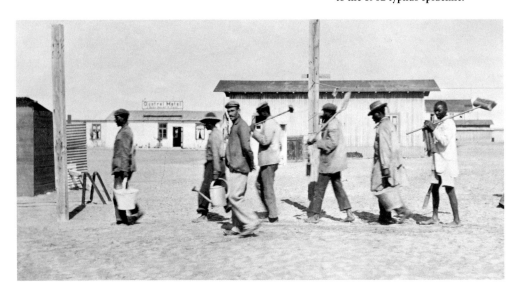

HOSPITAL FEVER

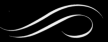

L ICE-BORNE *RICKETTSIA* becomes most lethal when it is present in large groups of people huddled close together. While the lice do not move far from a human host, scratching or restlessness will cause the creature to move about onto adjacent people. This is why it is also called "jail fever," "camp fever," "ship fever," and "war fever." These are all circumstances where people are confined in close quarters with low standards of hygiene.

Typhus was also known as "hospital fever" and that is where it was at its most lethal. Lice are very sensitive to temperature fluctuations in their host and as soon as a fever causes a temperature rise in the infected patient the lice will move away as quickly as possible to find a new host with a cooler core body temperature. All patients, whether hospitalized for broken limbs, dysentery, non-lethal ailments, or minor wounds, then become infected and that is why *Rickettsia* was able to decimate entire hospitals. An army on campaign would set up makeshift hospitals in filthy peasant houses, churches, or any other appropriate building, where those suffering from fevers were not separated from the other sick, leading to a crushing mortality rate. Of course, cold environments such as Russia in winter led to even more overcrowding and consequently even higher death rates.

Typhus was also common in the squalid environment of early prisons and asylums. Prisoners often huddled together in damp, filthy cells, allowing lice to spread easily. "Jail fever" was also known as "aryotitus fever" and such was its severity that being held over until trial could be a death sentence. Many women accused of witchcraft during the "great burning" of the 17th and 18th centuries never got to trial but died first.

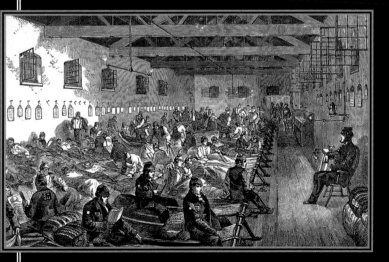

LEFT Prisons were perfect breeding grounds for typhus. It spread from these hotbeds of infection into the general population.

TYPHUS THE KINGMAKER

It is believed that Spanish soldiers may have caught typhus in Cyprus as they returned from the Crusades. The first large-scale outbreak of "war fever" or "camp fever," as it was known during this period, was when the Spanish army of Ferdinand and Isabella blockaded the Moors in Granada, their last stronghold on the Spanish mainland. The victorious monarchs had assembled an army of 25,000 crack fighters in 1489 and had realistic expectations that they would be able to clear the last Muslim outpost out of Spain.

Their grand plans were shattered when typhus decimated the army. Three thousand people died in combat, but 17,000 died of the disease. The symptoms described included fever, red spots over the arms, back and chest, followed by delirium, gangrenous sores, and the stink of rotting flesh.

The remnants fled, taking the new, deadly bacteria with them. Typhus became endemic in many pockets of Europe and would bide its time waiting until conditions were favorable to spread even farther.

Charles V of Spain was saved by typhus when the superior French army blockaded his 11,000 troops in Naples in 1527. Twenty-five thousand French soldiers died from camp fever. This reversed Charles's dire situation, allowing him to be crowned Holy Roman Emperor in 1530. All of Europe looked upon the deadly pestilence that obliterated the French army as an act of God.

Typhus changed history in many other instances. The Habsburg emperor Maximillian II had the Turks on the run and threatened Constantinople in the 1560s, but his army was cut down, allowing an Ottoman resurgence. Early campaigns against the Protestant heresy were terminated by the disease, allowing Protestantism to continue and ultimately leading to the devastating Thirty Years' War (1618–48).

The Black Assize

The virulence of typhus was demonstrated in the Black Assize at Oxford, England, in 1577, where the disease leaped from prisoners undergoing a trial and decimated the legal staff including the High Sherriff, the Sergeant at Arms, and even the judges. The Catholic bookbinder Rowland Jenks was being tried for distributing heretical books. His trial attracted a large audience that packed the smelly and stuffy courtroom. Jenks got off lightly: Although found guilty, he was only sentenced to have his ears cut off, no doubt to ensure that he did not hear any more "popish" propaganda. The audience was not so lucky. It was estimated that 500 people, including 100 staff from Oxford, came down with "spotted fever" during the next few weeks.

In 1759 it was reckoned that a quarter of all those imprisoned died of this malady. Scourge infected London's Old Bailey from adjacent Newgate Prison and killed a large number of court personnel including Sir Samuel Pennant, Lord Mayor of London, in 1750.

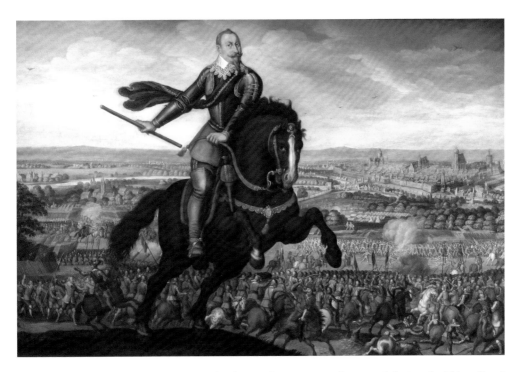

ABOVE **The Swedish King Gustavus Adolphus, hero of the Thirty Years' War, during which thousands died of typhus.**

Much of Central Europe was decimated during the Thirty Years' War, and while there are estimates that 350,000 soldiers died in battle, at least 10 million people died of other causes. Most of these died of typhus, which followed Protestant and Catholic armies as they marched back and forth across the blighted German landscape. One battle between Gustavus Adolphus and Baron von Wallenstein was prevented in 1632 when both armies lost a total of 18,000 men while camped in front of Nuremberg. It was this war that spread the contagion throughout Europe, allowing it to become entrenched in the population. Poland and Russia saw widespread epidemics and for the first time the bacterium entered France, taking a fearful toll of the new resistance-less population. Sixty thousand died in Lyon alone, and Burgundy was hard hit. Established throughout Europe, typhus waited for its next great chance. A diminutive Corsican with grand ambitions would grant the disease its next great triumph.

MUCH OF CENTRAL EUROPE WAS DECIMATED DURING THE THIRTY YEARS' WAR, AND WHILE THERE ARE ESTIMATES THAT 350,000 SOLDIERS DIED IN BATTLE AT LEAST 10 MILLION PEOPLE DIED OF OTHER CAUSES. MOST OF THESE DIED OF TYPHUS.

NAPOLEON'S GREATEST FOE

When Napoleon crossed the Neman River into the Russian Empire, there were upward of 320,000 men in his central army group. A short distance downstream Marshall Davout's veteran First Corps of 70,000 men also crossed into the Russian empire on June 24, 1812. The Grande Armée had taken almost a year to march to the frontier, the troops coming from every corner of the First Empire. It was the largest army mustered since Xerxes of Persia had invaded Greece. But none would return.

The campaign faced many obstacles. Once beyond the rich, settled agricultural lands of Central Europe, Napoleon's military machine began to break down. The Polish roads were not built to bear the heavy guns and, most importantly, the supply wagons needed to support his massive army. Consequently, Napoleon's supply trains came to a stop once they crossed the Neman River. The large carts with their half-ton loads of food and ammunition got bogged down and were left behind. Thanks to a shortage of feed, thousands of horses died after eating unripened rye (10,000 horses died on one day alone in early July). Napoleon had intended that his men would use the supplies on the wagons before consuming the livestock that pulled the wagons, but the animals died too soon, leaving the contents of the wagons to rot. The plan to use rivers as axes of supply also failed due to the dry winter.

Ignored Warnings

Contrary to some rather strongly worded advice from both his chief surgeon and support commanders, Napoleon decided to advance the main body of his army with as much haste as possible into Russia, leaving his supply trains to catch up on their own. Napoleon had been repeatedly warned by the surgeon that Poland had large endemic foci of typhus throughout the country and that the disease was rife among the peasants. As a consequence, orders were issued forbidding the soldiers to fraternize with the Polish citizenry under pain of death. These orders went largely unheeded, however, as the army, which rapidly ran out of food and supplies, began raiding nearby villages in search of food for its starving personnel. These forays inevitably brought the soldiers into contact with the Polish peasantry. This resulted in epidemic typhus being brought into the camps along with the returning troops. The consequences were disastrous. Over 80,000 French soldiers died in the first month of the epidemic. An abnormally hot summer had produced near-drought conditions in Poland prior to Napoleon's arrival. What scarce water was available was used for drinking, with bathing and clothes washing nearly impossible. In such an environment heavy infestations of body lice were inevitable. To make matters still worse, Poland was suffering from an abnormally cold winter in 1812, forcing the ill-prepared French soldiers to huddle together for warmth at night, facilitating the spread of typhus among themselves.

Decimator of Armies

Napoleon's Grande Armée began to evaporate before a shot had been fired. Even the well-provisioned Guard lost a third of its strength by the end of July. By August 17, Davout's 1st Corps was down to 35,000 men having lost 50 percent of its strength. Disease wasn't confined to the central column. The Second Corps to the north of the main thrust had lost 50 percent of its men after 36 days.

Typhus was not the only cause of death, but it factored largely in this horrendous rate of casualties. Convalescing soldiers were usually expected to rejoin their units after some rest and recuperation, but there was no effort made to separate different illnesses and a short stint in a field hospital often resulted in a deadly infection. The dead were not cremated but left to rot. Passing soldiers and peasants would take what items of clothing they required, so perpetuating the disease. Whole peasant families were found dead in their miserable dwellings, having died from typhus. Generals were in no doubt as to what was killing their men, reporting the "terrible epidemic" scything through their ranks. One German lieutenant wrote of the "variety of diseases, chief among them dysentery, ague, and typhus."

As usual it was blamed on miasma. One doctor in the French army offered the explanation that the illness "appeared spontaneously from the dirtiness of the clothes." Since they were on campaign, they could not change or wash their uniforms. He also attributed it to malnutrition, fatigue, and congestion. He presumed that the fact that large numbers of men were assembled together meant that it the illness became "more frequent and more serious." However, he attributed this to the putrid odors of rotting dead bodies lining the roads that they marched along. In one observation, at least, he was spot on: "Typhus began to stand out because it was so infectious."

Platoons were reduced to 16 men, regiments to a few hundred, and divisions to a thousand. Napoleon had raged at his ill-equipped surgeon, Dr. Larrey, but had nevertheless continued to Moscow. By September his Grande Armée was down to 125,000 men, only slightly larger than the Russian forces. When he faced the Russians at the Battle of Borodino on September 7, 1812, he could no longer dictate terms to them.

Even though the French army got to Moscow, the Russian Emperor Alexander I refused to concede defeat. He knew well the state of his enemy's troops, which by this time were reduced to 90,000 men. The great majority, possibly as high as 300,000, had died of epidemic typhus and dysentery. Actual combat losses amounted to less than 100,000. As the Grande Armée entered Moscow on September 14, they found that all the food stores had been burned by the Russians in order to make the critical food shortage of the French even worse.

Typhus didn't relax its grip on the French army in Moscow. Casualties from the Battle of Borodino were put into hospital with sufferers who had typhus. A slow stream of soldiers from the rear area were bundled into the few hospitals or into intact

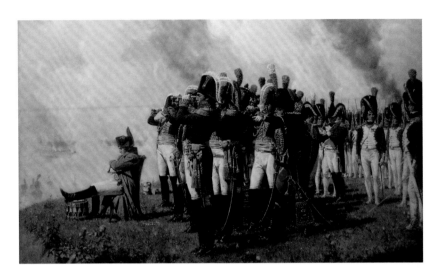

houses. The Foundling Hospital contained 1,850 men of whom 1,800 died from fever.

Doctors well knew the different stages of typhus and could have separated fever victims from other casualties, but in the chaos of the Grande Armée they had neither the time, space, nor resources. The wards stank of feces and urine, as well as the rotting flesh from suppurating wounds and gangrenous limbs. At night, typhus patients entered the delirium that preceded death, engaging in conversations with lost family members on the other side of the continent. Many had their eyes wide open as they gazed on imagined scenes of homes and loved ones. The signs of impending death increased. Raving tongues were covered with a thick, noxious film and teeth turned black as their eyes became sunken into their pale cheeks. Many began to cough uncontrollably as their lungs sought oxygen for the ravaged cardiovascular system. Others took short, shallow breaths. Some spasmed with "tendon jolts" as their arms and legs snapped into the air while others sought to throw off their clothes and bolted for the door before collapsing onto fellow patients. Many just stared dully into space before quietly expiring in a pool of their own urine and sweat. As life left the infected soldiers, so did their lice. They crawled off the bodies through the pestilent straw and as soon as they found a new warm body they started feeding again.

One Belgian doctor, De Kerckhove (Belgium was at the time part of greater France), wrote his observations of the journey the men followed before their death. They appeared to have a slow pulse and the face became puffy. Soon the "broken limb" phase set in where the patient became entirely listless and unable to make any but the smallest movement. Fever and chills followed, as well as a white film covering

ABOVE Napoleon invaded the Russian Empire with more than 550,000 men. By the Battle of Borodino he had lost more than half to starvation, thirst, and illness.

the tongue and an insatiable thirst. Vision, hearing, and the power of speech seemed to fade before insomnia and delirium set in. The small purplish spots so typical of the disease began to appear as well as larger subcutaneous hemorrhages.

Finally, just before death, the victims seemed to have some respite. The skin became cooler and they had some vestiges of energy. At night the bodies' systems crashed, they seemed to become lifeless corpses although still with a pulse, and gangrene spread particularly where tight clothes or vests hindered circulation. De Kerckhove did notice that some died almost immediately, as if the fatigues of the campaign had weakened them too much.

RETREAT!

Realizing that the war had been lost, Napoleon called for a full-scale retreat back to France. Many of the sick were bundled onto the remaining carts but, seeing them as deadweight, the drivers would drive over obstacles, causing their passengers to fall out of the cart to die by the roadside.

Once again the effect of typhus limited Napoleon's options. Seeking to take another route through fertile, unplundered territory, he tried to crash through the Russian army under Marshal Kutuzov in the Battle of Maloyaroslavets in October 1812. This route was denied him, again because he did not have enough reserves to break through, and the Grande Armée was forced to retreat along its previous route, which was entirely denuded of food and resources. What typhus had begun, the Russian winter, starvation, and enraged peasants finished.

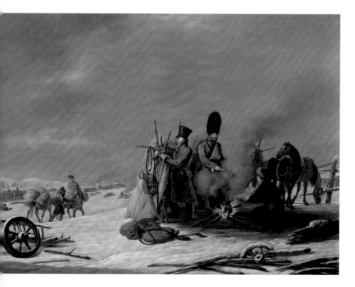

In later battles after the retreat from Moscow, typhus was an ever-present drain on the resources of Napoleon's military. In 1813 typhus spread through the newly raised army of conscripts and foreign levies. Napoleon managed to raise another Grande Armée of half a million men, but by the Battle of Leipzig in October

LEFT *Night Quarter to Molodetschno,* by Johannes Hari (1772–1849), depicts an episode from Napoleon's disastrous retreat from Russia.

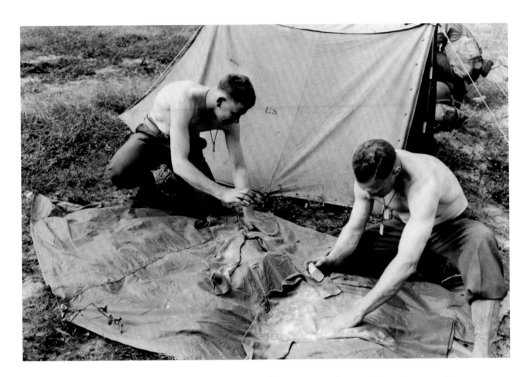

1813 his army had been reduced to 170,000 with the majority of casualties suffered through disease. It has been estimated that in 1813 he lost 217,000 to typhus, 7,000 died in Königsberg while 20,000 new recruits died in Dresden and Prussia before these areas were evacuated. The Russian army was not exempt and lost an estimated 70,000 men to typhus as they pursued the retreating French. Ten percent of the German civilian population were struck down, particularly in Saxony, where the economy and lands were devastated.

ABOVE DDT was used in World War II to fumigate uniforms. Here, American GIs dust their uniforms with the deadly powder.

After Napoleon was banished to St. Helena, another epidemic struck Europe between 1815 and 1819, and it is estimated to have had 37 percent mortality for those who were infected. In World War I typhus took a dreadful toll of soldiers on the Eastern Front, and Serbia was particularly hard hit in the first six months of the conflict, with at least 150,000 deaths. The invention of the insecticide DDT between the wars allowed lice to be cleaned from clothes, and a typhus vaccine was developed by Harold R. Cox in 1937. While not eliminating the disease, it did reduce its virulence. The prevalence of typhus is now much reduced due to the development of broad-spectrum antibiotics, against which *Rickettsia prowazekii* has no defense.

8

TROPICAL DISEASES

DURING THE COLONIAL PERIOD FROM 1500 to 1900, Europeans seized much of the world's landmass from its indigenous inhabitants. While many territories were temperate and benign, well suited to the European constitution, the tropics (the zone between the Tropic of Cancer in the north and the Tropic of Capricorn in the southern hemisphere) offered a host of nasty new diseases that decimated the new arrivals. These included yellow fever, dengue fever, and elephantiasis.

CROWD DISEASES IN THE COLONIES

Some Europeans were able to carve successful careers for themselves in the many colonies established between the 16th and 20th centuries. But for countless others it led to an early grave. Even the hardiest physical specimens were cut down in their prime. They were subject to a host of horrendous heirloom and crowd diseases to which the indigenous population had built up something of a resistance. In the 17th and 18th centuries it was possible for half the Europeans based in India to die of heat-stroke, fever, or other epidemics in a single year. Ninety percent of the British population of Bombay (now Mumbai) were wiped out in 1692. Six out of seven English servicemen in the early 19th century never returned home from India. Resistance had to be developed, but even those who survived bouts of fever were often prematurely aged and lacking in vigor.

As well as the new disease encountered in the hot and hostile tropical environment, the colonists had to deal with Old World sicknesses such as dysentery, typhoid, plague, and smallpox, which thrived in the unsanitary conditions found in the colonies. The most lethal was Asiatic cholera (covered in depth in chapter 9), which traveled through the colonies to ravage European populations. Nine out of ten sufferers died from this disease and the interval between the symptoms first emerging and death could be as

BELOW **The English began their expansion into the Indian subcontinent and were able to overcome military opposition. The real challenge was surviving tropical diseases.**

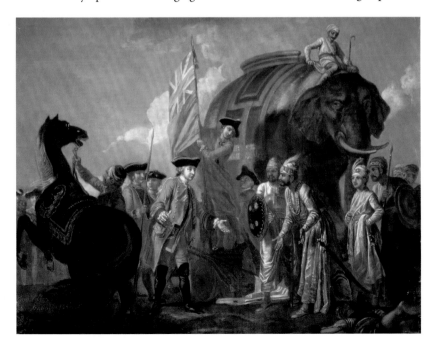

little as three hours. One member of the East India Company told of two instances when he had shared luncheon with fellow officers and buried them before tea.

The heat of the dry season in places such as India also contributed to the early mortality rate. Judges, soldiers, and administrators all had to "keep up appearances" in front of the "native" people and wear their full panoply of woolen western kit. Boils and carbuncles were prone to erupt and these too became vectors of infection.

The tropical diseases of Papua New Guinea were fierce enough to keep European settlers at bay for hundreds of years. Although first "discovered" by the Portuguese in 1526, it wasn't until the 1960s that the entire island was bought under European control. The lowlands weren't settled until the 1880s. One of the most ambitious colonies, which was founded under false pretensions as a new Garden of Eden by the French Marquis de Rays, saw 930 of the original 1,000 colonists die within three years. Papua was seen as such a hotbed of virulent diseases that only the German First Empire was interested in annexing it because all other likely colonial possessions had been snapped up by competing powers.

During the 1880s the Germans also colonized West Africa and Southeast Africa, another particularly lethal biosphere. Many military expeditions were ravaged by

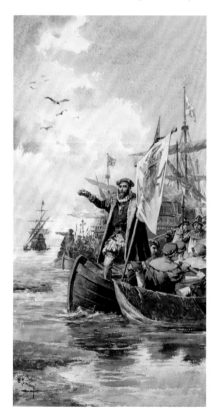

fever as well as native weapons, and one column of 120 soldiers operating in the Congo vanished and was never seen again. From the very first years of German colonialism in Africa, cholera, malaria, yellow fever, leprosy, and African trypanosomiasis were some of the tropical diseases that worried the colonial authorities, soldiers, merchants, missionaries, and colonists.

The high mortality rate in the German colonies led to several other problems. The lack of doctors in the colonies exacerbated the health problems encountered by settlers and it was often difficult to find Western experts who were willing to build infrastructure such as railroads. The filth, mosquitoes, and flies all contributed to the mortality rate of the early colonists. Most ailments could have been cured by penicillin, but by the time it became commonly used, most colonial powers were vacating their empires. One of the most lethal and mobile diseases was yellow fever.

LEFT **Vasco da Gama landed at Calicut (Kozhikode) in 1498. He opened up a route for Europeans to gain great wealth—if they could survive the new diseases.**

MOSQUITOES CARRY NEW and old diseases. Their means of transmitting diseases are as horrendous as they are common. Within their gut they can carry protozoa causing malaria, viruses such as chikungunya, and tiny worm-like filaments that cause filariasis, which can develop into elephantiasis. Perhaps the most revolting ailment mosquitoes carry is the larva of the human botfly. The female botfly glues its larvae onto the belly of a host mosquito. As the mosquito feeds the glue melts, discharging the maggots, which then begin burrowing into the skin of their new host.

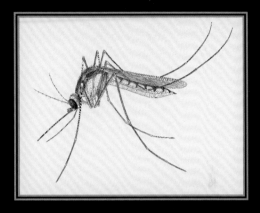

ABOVE **Specimens preserved in amber confirm that mosquitoes have been part of life on Earth for millions of years. Over time the species has evolved to carry many infectious organisms.**

Mosquitoes are particularly efficient at carrying any arbovirus (a virus carried by ticks, fleas, and mosquitoes) that has been able to enter the human population due to disruption and exploitation of the natural environment. Several of these diseases entered the human biosphere during the colonial era, the most notorious being yellow fever and dengue fever. These are both hemorrhagic fevers, and both were spread from their natural habitat in tropical West Africa. They have spread to humans because people altered their lifestyle and environments, thereby forcing the virus to adapt.

Monkeys living in the top level of the rainforest canopies of West Africa were the original carriers of yellow fever. It was carried by the mosquito *Aedes aegypti*, which originally bred in wet tree hollows. Through forest clearing the mosquito and its virus migrated into human communities where over generations the native population was able to develop resistance. Not so the new colonial overlords, who found the disease deadly in the extreme, and who carried it around the world in repeated patterns of infection. Dengue followed a similar trajectory and continues to evolve into new and deadly forms.

Mosquitoes also carry diseases that have thrived in human populations for millennia, including malaria. They also carry more recent killers such as West Nile virus and the recently discovered Zika virus, which was not identified until 1947. No vaccine is yet available for either of these diseases.

Yellow Fever

Yellow fever virus is named after the yellow skin resulting from jaundice, caused by the liver shutting down. The Spanish name *vomito negro* (black vomit) refers to the other major symptom, caused by internal bleeding particularly in the stomach and intestines. A crowd disease spread by various types of tropical and subtropical mosquitoes, the particular horror of yellow fever is engendered by its manner of dispersal. Populations on both sides of the Atlantic would be free of the disease for years and then seemingly out of nowhere, the disease would strike and cut a swathe through the population before again disappearing. This cycle began in the 16th century and lasted until the 19th century, causing untold suffering. The victims were not to know that the virus was communicated by mosquito bite. One infected person could join the community and, upon their being bitten, mosquitoes would spread the disease throughout the helpless community. Perhaps the worst aspect of the disease was the false hope it gave to sufferers. Afflicted individuals would rave deliriously but for a short window of time would become rational and lucid before dropping dead. Many well knew that the brief reprieve from delirium was the final moment they would be alive. Affected populations were able to notice that infections ceased as soon as cold weather occurred.

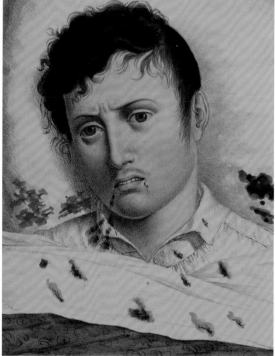

Yellow fever virus is mainly transmitted through the bite of infected yellow fever mosquitoes, but also by other aggressive mosquitoes such as the tiger mosquito. The virus is taken up by a female when she ingests the blood of an infected human or other primate. Reinfection occurs when another person is bitten. The viruses exit the bloodstream and head to the lymph nodes, where they replicate before moving to the kidneys; they then begin to kill the cells there, forming necrotic masses (dead tissue).

The first fever begins after an incubation period of three to six days. Most

LEFT **This patient is in the last stage of yellow fever. As his organs break down he vomits black bile and bleeds profusely.**

cases only cause a mild infection with fever, headache, chills, back pain, fatigue, loss of appetite, muscle pain, nausea, and vomiting. In these cases, the infection lasts only three to four days. In 15 percent of cases sufferers enter a second, toxic phase of the disease with recurring fever, this time accompanied by jaundice due to liver failure, as well as abdominal pain. Bleeding in the mouth, eyes, and gastrointestinal tract causes horrendous vomiting of blackened bile and blood. Depending on the virulence of the strain of virus or the degree of immunity, fatality rates for those infected before the 20th century were usually between 30 and 50 percent as the kidneys and other organs failed.

BELOW **Doctors were able to track the progress of yellow fever by examining the patient's tongue.**

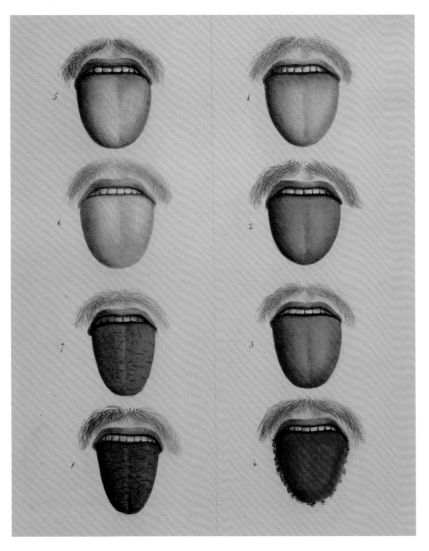

As well as hitting civilian populations in the new colonies, many military campaigns were frustrated by the ravages of yellow fever. In 1654 a French army was decimated as it sought to capture the Caribbean island of St. Lucia. In 1741 Admiral Edward Vernon lost half his fleet to an outbreak while attacking Spanish-held Colombia, and Napoleon Bonaparte's overseas ambitions were terminated when his French army was all but destroyed in 1803 while trying to reclaim Haiti.

At least 25 major outbreaks followed in North America, with the last major fatalities in 1905 in New Orleans. New Orleans had previously been hit in 1853, when corpses rotted in the streets as the gravediggers could not cope with the workload. Europe wasn't spared, since as travelers crisscrossed the Atlantic they often took the virus with them. In 1821 in Barcelona, Spain, thousands died.

Initially all kinds of causes were blamed. Some saw it as a contagious disease passed from person to person, while others blamed it on bad coffee or smelly oysters. It primarily attacked European settlers, especially newcomers, and African slaves seemed to be immune. No doubt as the disease originated in Africa, slaves had developed a greater degree of immunity over preceding generations, making them perfect workers for the swampy plantations in the New World.

Yellow Jack

The evolutionary origins of yellow fever most likely lie in East or Central Africa. It must have leaped the primate–human species divide and was spread between the continents—along with its host mosquito, *Aedes aegypti*—with the slave trade. Though it is not known when it first infected humans, the first reported outbreak of the disease was on the Caribbean island of Barbados in 1647. It was called "Barbados distemper"

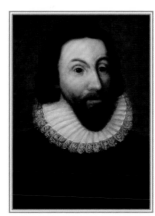

by Massachusetts governor John Winthrop, who instituted the first North American quarantine regulations to protect his colony from infection. Thenceforth, any ship with yellow fever on board would have to fly a yellow flag, hence the disease's other name of "Yellow Jack."

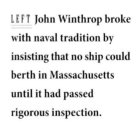

LEFT **John Winthrop broke with naval tradition by insisting that no ship could berth in Massachusetts until it had passed rigorous inspection.**

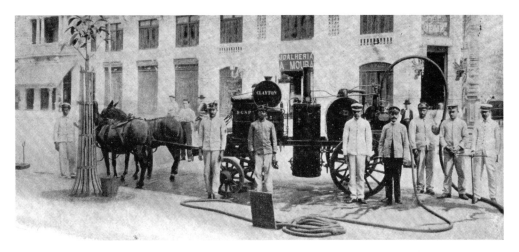

America's Frequent Visitor

Becoming endemic in the Americas, yellow fever became a frequent visitor to many communities where it made repeated appearances. Philadelphia's ravenous mosquitoes provided the perfect vehicle for spreading the disease in 1793 by first lunching on an infected victim and then biting a healthy one. The first fatalities appeared in July and the numbers grew steadily. The afflicted initially experienced pains in the head, back, and limbs accompanied by a high fever. These symptoms would often disappear, giving a false sense of security. Shortly, the disease would announce its return with an even more severe fever and turn the victim's skin a ghastly yellow while he vomited black clots of blood. Death soon followed as the victim slipped into a helpless stupor.

ABOVE Clayton disinfectors were used to saturate enclosed areas with sulfur gas to kill germs. Some were mounted on boats and used to sanitize dangerous cargoes.

One of the most frightening things about yellow fever was the rapidity with which it struck down its victims. An eyewitness to the 1793 Philadelphia outbreak wrote:

In private families the parents, the children, the domestics lingered and died, frequently without assistance. The wealthy soon fled; the fearless or indifferent remained from choice, the poor from necessity. The inhabitants were reduced thus to one-half their number, yet the malignant action of the disease increased, so that those who were in health one day were buried the next. The burning fever occasioned paroxysms of rage, which drove the patient naked from his bed to the street, and in some instances to the river, where he was drowned. Insanity was often the last stage of its horrors.

—SAMUEL BRECK, *QUOTED IN AMERICAN HISTORY TOLD BY CONTEMPORARIES (VOLUME III)*, ALBERT BUSHNELL HART (ED.), 1931

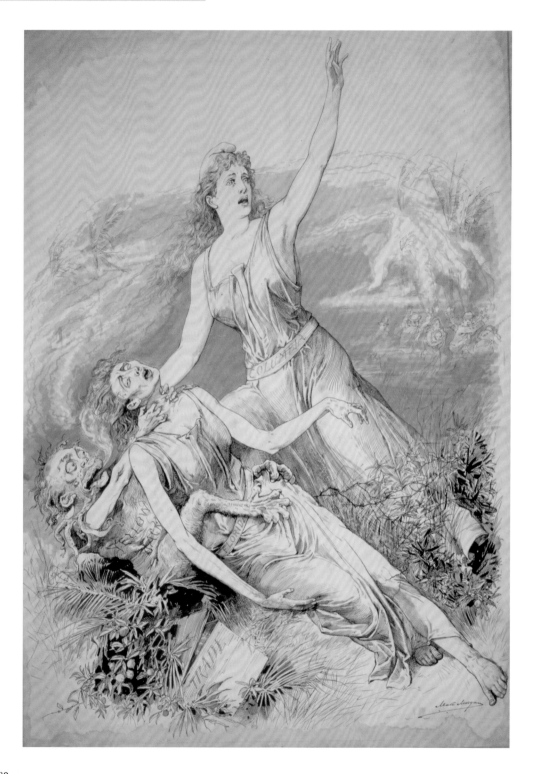

He also wrote an anecdote detailing its effect on one individual:

The poor man was then alive and begging for a drink of water. His fit of delirium had subsided, his reason had returned, yet the experience of the doctor enabled him to foretell that his death would take place in a few hours; it did so, and in time for his corpse to be conveyed away by the cart at the hour appointed. This sudden exit was of common occurrence. The whole number of deaths in 1793 by yellow fever was more than four thousand.

—SAMUEL BRECK (IBID)

Pensacola, Florida, gives a terrific example of how successions of epidemics struck certain localities. After an initial visitation the virus returned repeatedly to kill the young who had not developed an immune response from a previous epidemic. Once an individual was infected and survived, they had lifelong immunity. This was of course not hereditary, and younger generations would be particularly hard hit.

The first major outbreak in Pensacola occurred in 1822 and many fled the disease. The population was reduced from 4,000 to about 1,400. The local council moved to a farm 15 miles (24 km) out of town to pass laws. The community seemed to recover but another epidemic in 1874 killed a third of the town's residents. In the erroneous belief that the disease was usually transmitted by day, victims were buried in the cemetery at night by the light of lanterns. This was the worst possible practice as the *Aedes aegypti* mosquito that transmits yellow fever generally bites at night. Commodore Melancthon Woolsey believed that rum was a tonic against contracting the fever. One day his servant forgot the rum and the poor commodore died soon after—an antiplacebo if you will.

By 1905 the link between the mosquito-borne virus and the disease had been identified. An incipient epidemic of 1905 was quickly brought under control by vigorously eradicating mosquitoes and by isolating victims under mosquito netting to prevent transmission of the virus from victims to mosquitoes.

Yellow Fever Today

A vaccine has been developed for yellow fever, but new vectors that can transmit the disease have been discovered as more jungle is penetrated, meaning that it is still a real threat in many impoverished nations. The best method to safeguard populations is to remove still water in the urban environment to make it more difficult for mosquitoes to breed, as well as maintaining vaccination programs. Currently there are 200,000 reported cases every year with a 15 percent mortality rate. Once the disease takes hold, hospitalization with rehydration and pain relief is the best that can be done.

LEFT **American authorities knew that yellow fever came from overseas imports. Here, "Yellow Jack" has escaped from a box of fruit to seize and kill.**

DENGUE FEVER

Related to yellow fever, dengue is not as deadly but it inflicts staggering pain and suffering on its victims. It begins with a sudden onset of fever followed by vomiting and a rash, as well as migraine-like pains behind the ears, and lower back pain. Severe cramping and muscular pain rotate around the body, being particularly severe in the head, back, and limbs.

Dengue fever, like yellow fever, is spread mainly by the mosquito *Aedes aegypti*. When a mosquito carrying dengue virus bites a person, the virus enters the skin together with the mosquito's saliva. It binds to and enters white blood cells and reproduces inside the cells while they move throughout the body. The white blood cells respond by producing a number of signaling proteins that are responsible for many of the symptoms, such as the fever, the flu-like illness, and the severe pains. In severe infections, virus production inside the body is greatly increased, and many more organs such as the liver and bone marrow are affected.

BELOW Fumigation is necessary in tropical climates, such as Mumbai, India, to kill mosquito populations that carry dengue fever.

In more severe cases dengue fever morphs into dengue hemorrhagic fever, which can be fatal. Fluid from the bloodstream leaks through the walls of small blood vessels into body cavities and as a result, less blood circulates in the blood vessels, and the blood pressure becomes so low that it cannot supply sufficient blood to vital organs. Furthermore, dysfunction of the bone marrow leads to reduced numbers of platelets,

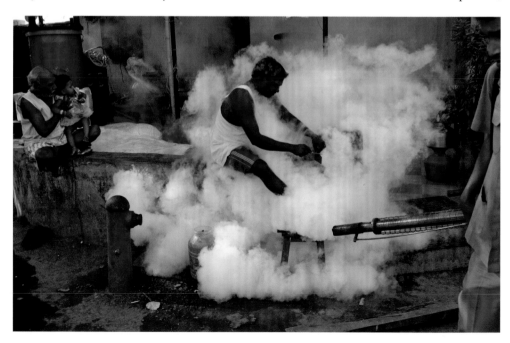

which are necessary for effective blood clotting; this increases the risk of bleeding, the other major complication of dengue. Fevers and a breakdown in the circulatory system lead to death.

Another disease brought from its motherland of Africa, dengue fever was probably carried to America and the Caribbean with the slave trade in the 16th century. Dengue fever was given a range of names all describing the unpleasant symptoms inflicted upon sufferers. Benjamin Rush, a founding father of the American Republic, called it "breakbone fever," because of the extreme cramps that were so painful, sufferers were sure their bones were bending and snapping. The Swahili term *ka dinga pepo* describing a sudden cramp-like seizure sent by an evil spirit is one possible origin of the word *dengue*, or else it may be a corruption of the term "dandy," describing the mincing walk produced by stiffening of limbs.

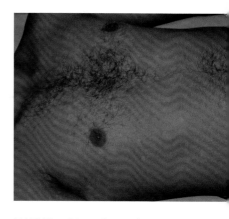
ABOVE The white rashes on this man's torso indicate that he is recovering from dengue fever.

The first large-scale outbreaks of dengue fever occurred in the 1780s as the host mosquito *Aedes aegypti* established itself in new habitats following colonial settlements. Dengue struck in Asia, Africa, North America, and tropical areas throughout the Pacific.

In 1906 the virus was isolated and in the early 20th century measures were taken to control the introduced *A. aegypti* with DDT. However, the growth of urbanized settlement throughout Asia and the associated lack of sewer facilities have led to a recent resurgence of dengue fever.

Dengue Fever Today

The most recent strain of dengue fever is a vicious killer. It first attacked luckless sufferers during the 1950s in Southeast Asia and the Philippines. Dengue hemorrhagic fever (DHF) leads to massive internal bleeding combined with agonizing muscle spasms and the combined symptoms lead to dengue shock syndrome, which results in coma and death in 15 percent of sufferers. It now runs rampant through the Asian Pacific and has even hit the Caribbean where in 1981 Cuba experienced 350,000 cases. The new disease is almost impossible to eradicate because there are currently at least four lethal strains, none of which bestows resistance on infected individuals. Its spread has been aided by the emergence of a new carrier. *Aedes albopictus*, the Asian tiger mosquito, is an aggressive feeder that swarms on its victims during the day, attacking any warm-blooded animal. Such is its ferocity that in some cities, parks and gardens are deserted as people literally flee the aggressive attacks of large voracious packs of these striped feeders.

ELEPHANTIASIS TROPICA

The means by which people contract *Elephantiasis tropica* is once again mosquitoes, which deliver a deadly package to unsuspecting victims. Only in this case, it is neither a virus nor a bacterium, but a tiny thread-like parasitic round worm, filaria, and its microscopic larvae, microfilariae. The larvae are left on the skin after the mosquito bite and they then bore into the new host and travel via the lymphatic system into the lymph nodes, where they proceed to breed so vigorously that the lymphatic system shuts down. The lymphatic system is crucial for the smooth running of any mammalian organism and is a complex system of lymphatic vessels, capillaries, and lymph nodes. It carries a clear, watery substance—lymph—which takes nutrients to cells and collects impurities, which it delivers to the lymph nodes. The lymphatic system's primary function is to drain impurities and harmful components from cells and tissues, and it uses muscle contractions to move the fluids and allow them to be expelled. The tiny worms set up "nests" within the lymphatic system, thus impeding the flow, causing chronic lymphedema (buildup of fluid) in the affected limbs. These symptoms can include grossly distorted arms and legs, and testicles that swell up until each is the size of a basketball. Toxins and impurities then build up and reduce the ability of the body's immune system to fight back.

RIGHT **In this illustration from 1614, the girl's lymphatic system has been infested with worm-like filariae, leading to a buildup of fluid in her lower limbs.**

BELOW **Legs, arms, and even testicles become grossly swollen when a person is infected with *Elephantiasis tropica*.**

There are three types of worms that can infect humans, all with their own particularly unpleasant symptoms. They are all spread by mosquitoes that feed on one infected person, then spread the disease as they feed on multiple other people within a community. The most common threadworm is *Wuchereria bancrofti*; infection leads to abnormal swelling in the genitals, breasts, arms, and legs. The other types of worm are *Brugia malayi* and *B. timori*. As well as the classic sign of elephantiasis—swollen limbs and underlying tissue—the skin thickens and begins to resemble elephant hide with many cracks and crevices, as well as dry, flaky eczema-like symptoms. This results from infestations where filariae located within the epidermis continue to breed, forming nodules of young worm colonies living among dead skin. Initial symptoms are fever chills and small nodules breaking out on the skin. Heavily infested people have incurable sores and severe abdominal pain, as the worms move out of the lymphatic system and infest subcutaneous fat and internal organs. The urine also becomes cloudy as lymph is often passed.

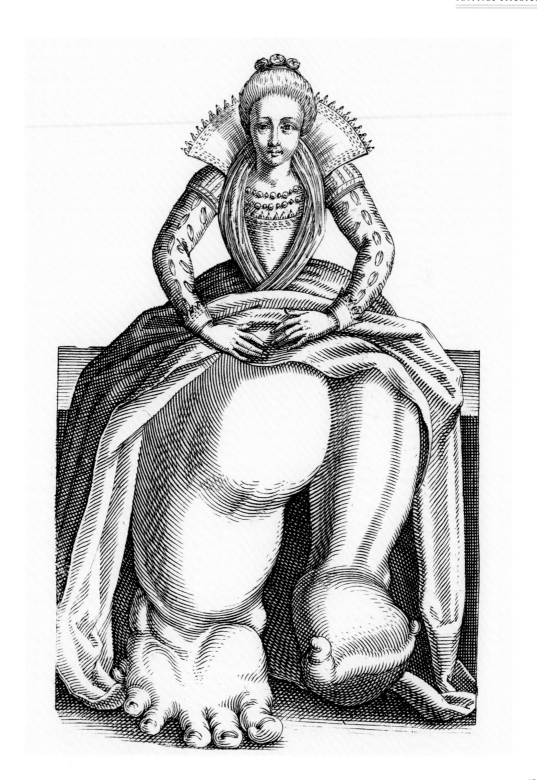

Lymphatic filariasis has existed in human populations from the dawn of history and early records indicate a familiarity with the condition. One of the earliest known records is an illustration of a client king and his wife in the tomb of Queen Hatshepsut of Egypt (1501–1480 BCE). The king of Punt's wife is clearly depicted with the swollen limbs characteristic of elephantiasis. A statue of Pharaoh Mentuhotep II depicts his swollen limbs, showing that not only the poor suffered. In 1100 BCE, during the time of Ramses II, a priest called Natsef-Amun died, and a recent autopsy of his mummified corpse revealed the abundant presence of filarial worms. In 600 BCE ancient Hindu doctors described the symptoms, and in Greek literature a clear distinction was drawn between the lesions associated with this disease and those seen in leprosy. The disease was quite common in ancient Japan and one woodcut depicts a man carrying his testicles in a sling supported by a pole.

The disease first impacted on Europeans when Tomé Pires, a Portuguese envoy to Goa, wrote in 1515:

> *Many people in Malabar, Nayars as well as Brahmans and their wives—in fact about a quarter or a fifth of the total population, including all the people of the lowest castes—have very large legs, swollen to a great size; and they die of this, and it is an ugly thing to see. They say that this is due to the water through which they go, because the country is marshy. This is called pericaes in the native language, and all the swelling is the same from the knees downward, and they have no pain, nor do they take any notice of this infirmity.*
> —THE SUMA ORIENTAL OF TOMÉ PIRES, TOMÉ PIRES, 1515, TRANS. ARMANDO CORTESAO, 1944

An Englishman wrote in his book *Ralph Fitch: England's Pioneer to India and Burma*: "This bad water causeth many of the people to be like lepers, and many of them have their legs swollen as big as a man in the waste [waist], and many of them are scant able to go."

Barbados Leg

As it took so long for symptoms to appear, Europeans at first seemed unaffected by elephantiasis. However, a virulent form took hold in expatriate populations in the West Indies and many plantation owners suffered what was called "Barbados leg."

As with many of these mysterious diseases that seemed to strike out of nowhere, all sorts of causes were blamed for elephantiasis. Rotten coconut milk, snake venom, bad water, and eating rotten fish were all suspected as culprits. Perhaps the most outlandish cause was the belief that sufferers were descendants of the murderers of St. Thomas the apostle, who traveled to India where he was killed.

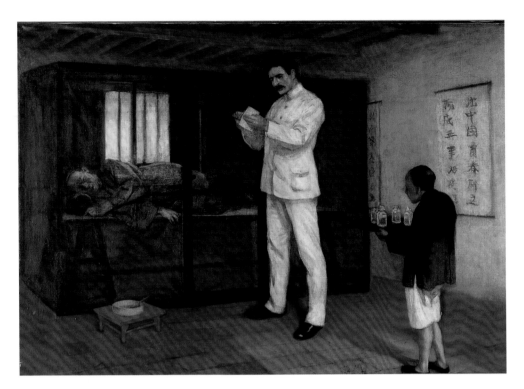

The Dutch explorer Jan van Linshoten saw whole villages that were infected with Barbados leg. Men, women, and children all seemed to be afflicted. He presumed that they were all born with the complaint due to the sins of their ancestors. A more plausible cause was described by Ralph Fitch, who wrote of the "knats which never ceased tormenting us" in areas where this debilitating disease was common.

ABOVE Patrick Manson was the first to realize that mosquitoes carried the lethal filariae.

Discovering the Cause

The mystery of the cause of this and similar diseases caused by microfilariae was finally solved in 1877 by Patrick Manson, a Scottish physician working in China. He noticed that his gardener had the worms in his blood, and placed the poor fellow within a mosquito-proofed room. He introduced uninfected bugs into the room to suck the gardener's blood and captured them in a wine glass before knocking them out with tobacco smoke. Upon dissection he found the worm in its larval stage and became the first to demonstrate conclusively the insect-borne transmission of any disease. He went on to earn fame and fortune, but the fate of his gardener is not, of course, recorded.

Lymphatic filariasis continues to be a threat to millions of people worldwide in 85 countries, and currently at least 120 million people are infected with the parasite.

At least 40 million are disabled or disfigured. The basic problem remains how to control the mosquito population. An infected person can be treated with a range of chemotherapy medicines which, while they do not kill the adult parasites, eliminate immature worms and reduce infection rates in local populations.

MALARIA

While not a charismatic or high-profile disease like yellow fever, where the symptoms were bound to grab the attention of early media and citizens alike, malaria has a range of symptoms that vary between each infected individual, making it initially quite hard to recognize. Some sufferers could live for years with mild, recurring bouts, while others would be carried off in a matter of days.

The earliest Western reference to malaria was by Hippocrates in the early 4th century BCE when he categorized malarial fevers as "quotidian" (occurring every day), "tertian" (every second day), and "quartan" (every third day).

Malaria was probably one of the original diseases to give rise to miasmic theory. Communities living near low-lying wet areas or stagnant pools were particularly susceptible to malarial infection as these were perfect breeding grounds for mosquitoes. Large sections of the Italian peninsula were mostly deserted even at the height of the Roman Empire due to malarial infestations. The word "malaria" is in fact derived from the Italian word *mal'aria* (bad air) and was first introduced into the English language in 1740 by Horace Walpole, the fourth Earl of Orford. Other names for malaria that have echoed through the centuries include "ague," "swamp fever," "malignant fever," "the shakes," and "Roman fever."

The disease resulting from the bite of an infective female *Anopheles* mosquito undoubtedly has infected the human genome for hundreds of thousands of years and is still a clear and present danger infecting at least half a billion people across the globe. In 1880

LEFT **Malaria remains a scourge in many parts of the world. This woman, painted in the 1930s, is suffering an episodic attack.**

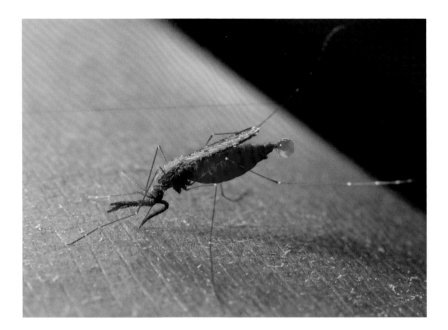

Charles Louis Alphonse Laveran, a French army surgeon, first recognized the malaria parasite in the blood of a soldier, but after one and a half centuries malaria is still a scourge killing millions of people every year. The reason malaria is so successful is that there are 60 species of the mosquito genus *Anopheles* and four species of the protozoan parasite that infects humans. *Plasmodium falciparum*, *P. vivax*, *P. ovale*, and *P. malariae* are all carried in the gut of the plethora of mosquito species, making it impossible to eradicate or even control all of the vectors of infection. If an infected person is bitten by a mosquito, the mosquito becomes infected too, able to transmit the infection to any further hosts that it feeds off.

ABOVE The *Anopheles* mosquito is just one genus of many that carry malaria. They transmit the infection from person to person by biting.

Plasmodium vivax and *P. falciparum* cause the most infections. Infections caused by *P. vivax* and *P. ovale* are relatively benign and can remain dormant within a host for years. *Plasmodium falciparum* is absolutely deadly and was chiefly responsible for killing colonizers and those people they colonized.

While they differ in intensity, the symptoms of all malarial infections can include a slowly rising temperature that then oscillates rapidly, causing chills interspersed with fever. Headaches, nausea, sweating, diarrhea, and anemia then ensue. It is this latter symptom that causes the yellow pallor that is an immediately recognizable side effect of the disease.

Malarial parasites are carried by the female *Anopheles* mosquito, which is commonly active at dusk and early evening. When an infected mosquito bites a human, the parasites roam in the bloodstream for around one hour before entering the liver and multiplying. Like a killer lurking in an alleyway, they remain hidden in the liver before the parasites return to the bloodstream; they then invade and multiply inside red blood cells until they burst. The released parasites then invade fresh red blood cells, causing the catalog of ills listed above. Chronic long-term sufferers experience these symptoms on a regular basis, as the parasites repeatedly leave the liver before entering the bloodstream and invading red blood cells, where they multiply furiously before bursting out of the cells to infect others.

Infections can be characterized as mild, chronic, or fatal. Those luckless colonizers infested by *Plasmodium falciparum* usually died as the symptoms escalated into a whole range of life-threatening conditions. Any small injuries became deadly hemorrhages, as blood was unable to clot. The red blood cells also died early, leading to a lack of oxygen being carried to organs; this resulted in the spleen, kidneys, and liver shutting down.

Many eyewitness accounts tell of the despair Europeans felt as their loved ones progressed to a painful death as pulmonary edema took hold. The breakdown in the circulatory system led to the lungs filling with fluid. Patients had extreme difficulty in breathing and an overwhelming feeling of suffocating or drowning, even while fully conscious. As they wheezed and gasped for breath they were racked by

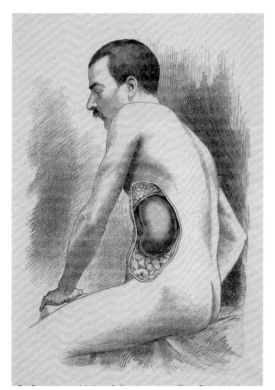

intense chest pains and severe palpitations, while they coughed out frothy sputum. These symptoms were made worse if they lay down and many had to sit up, gazing into their loved ones' eyes as they slowly suffocated to death. Sleep was almost impossible and patients stacked on weight as fluids built up while the heart desperately tried to pump blood into the extremities.

Cerebral malaria often occurred, where the illness penetrated the cranium leading to high fevers, severe headaches, drowsiness, delirium, coma, and death.

LEFT **An enlarged spleen is a typical symptom of malarial infection. Until the 1930s the only effective treatment was the drug quinine, an alkaloid extracted from the cinchona tree.**

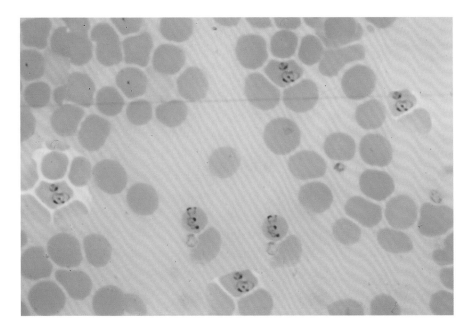

ABOVE **A close study of blood**
reveals the presence of the
malaria parasite when it
emerges from the liver.

Where Does Malaria Come From?

Malaria has been on the Earth millions of years before humans walked the planet. Ancient malaria parasites were found in the gut of mosquitoes preserved in amber during the Paleogene period (66–23 million years ago) and have been dated as at least 30 million years old. It has been suggested that malaria evolved in Africa and over the ages was able to adapt into different lineages, specifically primates, birds, rodents, and reptiles. *Plasmodium falciparum* probably originated in gorillas while *P. vivax* most likely came from chimpanzees and gorillas. One of the lesser forms, *P. knowlesi*, appears to have transferred in limited numbers to humans from the Asian macaque monkeys, while *P. malariae* is specific to humans and cannot survive in any other carriers.

Genetic markers affecting blood types in selected human populations indicate that humans began to develop resistance to malaria during the Neolithic Revolution. Acting as a crowd disease against a sedentary population, malaria-carrying mosquitoes were able to feast on early farmers living in one area and requiring constant water supplies, whereas the earlier nomadic peoples could avoid "pestilential miasma" and move after alternative food sources. Some genetic defenses were built up in selected Mediterranean populations and also in southeast Asian groupings. Populations from temperate Northern European climates did not have the opportunity to develop these defenses, and this made them extremely vulnerable once they occupied tropical and subtropical empires.

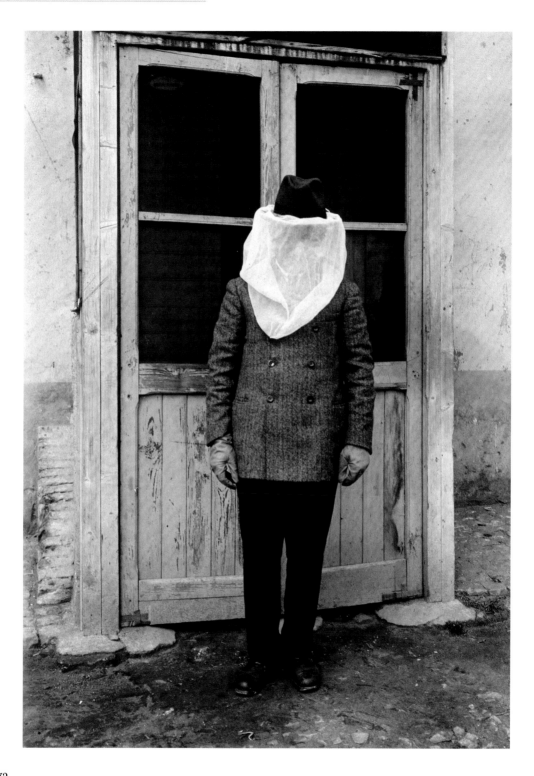

The earliest textual reference describing likely symptoms is contained in the Chinese medical classic *Nei Ching*, dated to 2700 BCE. Ancient Egyptians were acutely aware of the dangers of mosquitoes and their laborers were given copious amounts of garlic (thought to repel the insects) from as early as the 3rd century BCE. Wealthier Egyptians, including Cleopatra, used more practical mosquito nets while sleeping. Molecular evidence from Egypt confirms the disease from at least 800 BCE.

Classical Greece was hard hit by malaria and it is likely that a particularly virulent strain hit the scattered populations of many city-states during the 4th century BCE. Hippocrates of Kos first ascribed the illness to *miasma* (Greek for pollution), and presumed the illness was caused by dangerous fumes emanating from the ground and spread by winds. Malaria became the prototype for a multiplicity of diseases blamed on foul air, and this theory became accepted wisdom right up until the 19th century. Hippocrates noted that the disease was most prevalent around foul-smelling and stagnant marshes and swamps. He was right in believing the disease emanated from these locations, he just didn't realize that mosquitoes were the carriers.

The Campagna region of southern Italy was renowned for its tough warriors who combined Latin steadfastness, Greek sophistication, and Oscan doggedness during the 5th to 2nd centuries BCE. This area was also known for a particularly nasty strain of malaria that depopulated large regions by attacking the liver and spleen. Not only the Campagna but also the Po Valley, the Pontine Marshes, and the Mezzogiorno region in the south were prey to the pestilence, until it was largely eliminated when

LEFT **The swamplands of southern Italy were made uninhabitable by the prevalence of malaria. This Italian from Nettuno protects himself with mosquito netting.**

BELOW **A 19th-century lithograph extolling the level of protection offered by mosquito nets.**

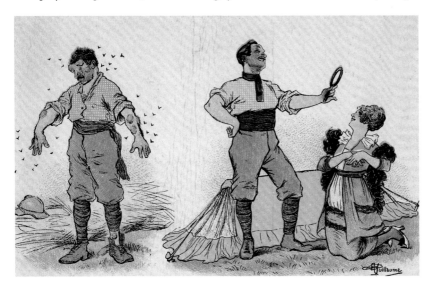

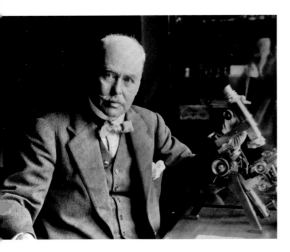

ABOVE **By examining hundreds of mosquitoes under the microscope, Ronald Ross was able to prove that they were the source of malaria.**

BELOW RIGHT **Quinine sulfate was an effective preventative against malaria. Issued to soldiers fighting in Burma during World War II, it was famous for turning those who imbibed it yellow.**

Mussolini's fascist regime drained many of these wetlands in the 1930s.

Between the 16th and the 18th centuries the slave trade and colonization of the Americas transported the more deadly *P. falciparum* to the New World. It added to the catalog of woes experienced by the indigenous population, but also exacted a terrible toll on the white settlers.

Benin in Africa was considered by many to be the most lethal hotspot for "the shakes." A ditty popular among mariners ran, "Beware the Blight of Benin, for there's one that comes out for every ten that goes in." The coasts and rivers of West Africa were particularly deadly and Benin was known as "The White Man's Grave." The English military were decimated with losses of up to 50 percent. In India at least 1.3 million people died every year as a result of malaria.

The Quest for a Cure

A British army doctor based in India, Ronald Ross (1857–1932), dissected hundreds of mosquitoes until he found the malaria parasite in the belly of a mosquito that had recently fed on an infected patient, finally proving the link between mosquitoes and malaria in 1897.

One common cure was to eat whole spiders cooked in butter. A more practical medicine is quinine, which was initially derived from the bark of the cinchona tree in South America. This drug attacks the parasite in the body and was used from the 17th century through to the 19th century. Currently vaccines are being developed, but none have been released commercially. In the mid-20th century malaria cases dropped dramatically with the widespread use of DDT sprayed over their breeding grounds. Obvious environmental issues arose with this program and the use of the highly toxic DDT is now banned. The best preventative is a good mosquito net.

Today about half of the world's population are at risk of contracting malaria. In 2015 there were more than 200 million reported cases and almost half a million deaths caused by the parasite. Sub-Saharan Africa is still the most affected area and accounts for 9 out of 10 malaria deaths.

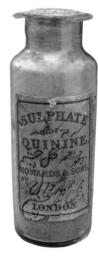

Yaws

Yaws is a particularly nasty disease, where a "mother pustule" forces its way to the surface of the skin before bursting. The initial infection then dries up and seems to disappear, but its disgusting job is done. The spirochete bacterium that causes the disease spreads over the skin and into the system and a whole range of nasty, painful "daughter yaws" rise up. These secondary lesions may be wart-like and similar to the "mother yaw," or may fill with pus before bursting. This disease is still endemic throughout Asia, the South Pacific, and Africa. Contact with fluids from a leaking lesion readily infects other victims, entering the bloodstream through minor cuts or abrasions. The yaws then spread over large portions of the skin before entering a tertiary stage where bones and joints become infected, leading to internal corruption, bleeding, and necrotic flesh. Cartilage rots out, and noses, in particular, can be disfigured after many years of active infection. They often become lopsided and in extreme cases rot away altogether. Lesions can develop into permanent callused carbuncles on the soles of the feet and the palms of the hands,

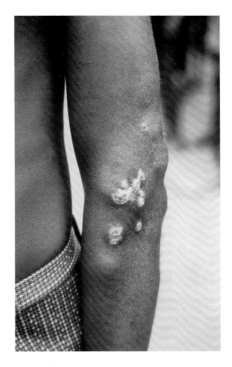

ABOVE **Yaws is transmitted when one of the lesions bursts and another person comes into contact with the resulting pus.**

which are referred to as "crab yaws," no doubt because this condition causes the hands and feet to contract into club-like appendages with little suppleness or movement.

The causative bacterium is *Treponema pallidum pertenue* and is related to syphilis. One form of syphilis can be transmitted through external contact with an infected person, by sharing cooking utensils, and through saliva; it does not need to be sexually transmitted. This form tends to be slightly more benign than sexually transmitted syphilis, and it doesn't always progress to the tertiary stage. Yaws is also related to *pinta*, another skin disease that leads to small bluish-black spots that clear up relatively quickly.

The first reference to yaws may come from the Bible where symptoms are mentioned along with plagues and pests. Similar bacteria have been found in primate species, and humans have been inoculated using primate antibodies. Yaws may have been present in primate populations up to 5 million years ago, before *Homo sapiens* diverged from their ape cousins.

Superstitions abounded in communities struck by yaws, and it was suggested that fish sauce should be avoided as well as astringent fruit. A single shot of penicillin is more effective and is almost 100 percent guaranteed to avoid a relapse. Yaws still remains a threat, particularly for children aged between 10 and 15 months, in poorer tropical and subtropical regions around the world. Attempts to eradicate the disease have failed, largely due to political instability.

LEISHMANIASIS

Leishmaniasis is a parasitic disease that is found in parts of the tropics, subtropics, and southern Europe. It is caused by infection with *Leishmania* parasites, which are spread by the bite of phlebotomine sandflies, or by coming in contact with other infected people and human waste. There are three forms of the disease. Cutaneous leishmaniasis causes open sores on the limbs and torso. Mucocutaneous leishmaniasis primarily attacks the mucous membranes and eats away the nose and mouth. Visceral leishmaniasis leads to fevers and can damage internal organs.

The most common form is cutaneous leishmaniasis, the symptoms of which are open circular wounds where the skin rots away, leaving unsightly open sores. However, these cutaneous sores can clear up, just leaving scarring. Much worse is the mucocutaneous form, in which parasites invade the mucous membranes of the nose, mouth, and throat, leading to extreme pain when breathing, eating, swallowing, or talking. The lesions develop under the skin leading to gross facial distortions, which can result in the poor sufferer being shunned by society. The visceral form enters the digestive tract,

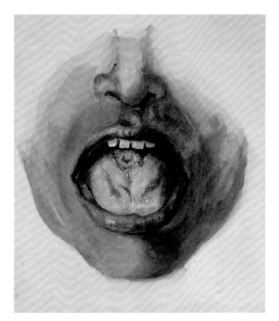

leading to gross swelling in the abdomen and death through anemia within a couple of years.

Descriptions of this disease first appear on tablets from the reign of King Ashurbanipal of Assyria from the 7th century BCE, which drew on information supplied as early as 2500 BCE. In India physicians called the disease *kala-azar*, meaning "black fever," or *dum dum* fever from a region near Calcutta (Kolkata). Spanish colonists referred to it as "valley sickness." In the Americas, evidence of the cutaneous form of the disease in Ecuador

LEFT **Sores resulting from leishmaniasis can appear anywhere on the body. This is a gangrenous lesion on the tongue.**

and Peru appears in pre-Inca pottery depicting skin lesions and deformed faces dating back to the 1st century. The disease was also known as "white leprosy" and it took a fearful toll on many colonists, the sores often acting as gateways for other more serious infections. One English plantation owner in the Caribbean counted 200 of these unsightly painful sores on one of his slaves and whipped the poor fellow, as he was in such pain that he was unable to work.

Today some medicines, including a range of antifungal and antibiotic treatments, are available for treatment of the disease but it still takes a severe toll and up to 50,000 deaths occur every year. It is currently found in most equatorial countries. The most effective treatment remains preventative measures such as chemically treated mosquito nets.

RIVER BLINDNESS

A European settler in Africa might have noticed a tiny black fly biting him and swatted it away. He would not know it, but that seemingly insignificant bite would cause unremitting pain, itchiness so intense that many were driven to suicide; others became blind. Most European colonists in subtropical Africa during the 19th century grabbed the fertile land adjacent to river valleys, not realizing that this was the preferred habitat of the female black fly *Simulium*. This aggressive fly could cause great discomfort as it attacked in swarms, biting any exposed flesh. Any short-term discomfort was nothing to the problems caused by a hitchhiker in the fly's gut—the filarial worm *Onchocerca volvulus*.

The flies impacted the human biosphere in Africa to a tremendous degree. Farmers seeking arable land would move to the riversides to plant their crops, but the devastating effects of river blindness would force whole communities into less fertile uplands, leading to unsustainable land clearing and successively poor harvests. Population pressure would force them back to the river valleys, where an individual could be expected to be bitten at least 20,000 times a year.

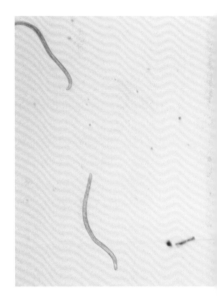

ABOVE The microfilaria *Onchocerca volvulus* is capable of overwhelming the body's defenses, resulting in a horrific death.

The first symptom of infection was intense itching caused by small communities of the worm breeding and living just under the surface of the skin. These worms could be clearly seen as they wriggled, twisted, curled, and coiled beneath the skin. Sufferers were driven to distraction and would resort to any means to try and stop the intense itching, which was referred to as *kru kru* in the local dialect. Some scraped off skin with knives and stones, while for some it was too much and they committed suicide.

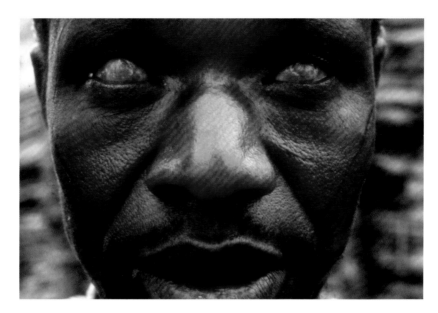

ABOVE **One of the final symptoms is blindness as the eyeball fills with dead and dying microfilaria parasites. This man is in his mid-thirties.**

The worms thrive in small nodules in the skin and lay up to 1,000 eggs per day. These larval worms then migrate to other spots on the skin as well as to the eyes to set up new colonies. Uninfected flies then suck blood from the infected person and transmit the disease to another person during their next meal.

The agonizing itching is partly caused by the body's natural inflammatory response to foreign organisms as it tries to expel the 100,000 dead or dying microfilariae produced each day in heavily infected people. A carrier can continue to transmit the disease for up to 15 years.

Colonists noticed other side effects. Skin lesions became common and the local people developed "leopard skin" as their lower limbs became discolored. The skin became less elastic as pustules containing millions of dead worms rotted and calcified, and the testicles became enlarged and pendulous. The final symptom was blindness, as fluid within the eyes became clogged with dead and dying minuscule worms. A slow and horrible death was the inevitable end for these sufferers.

River Blindness Today

River blindness is now much less prevalent. In the 1970s and 1980s the WHO (World Health Organization) began the Onchocerciasis Control Program. This is a three-pronged strategy, which involves spraying larvicides in local waterways, treating infected people with the drug ivermectin, and providing strategies so locals can avoid being bitten. These include being less active at the time of day when the flies are more likely to be engaged in feeding.

Sleeping Sickness

If one disease seemed destined to stop European colonization of Africa, it was the "sleepy distemper," now known as sleeping sickness or African trypanosomiasis. Not only did it attack natives and settlers, but it also wiped out introduced herds of cattle and horses. Early explorers such as David Livingstone (1813–73) noticed that any horses, oxen, or dogs accompanying his expeditions were doomed to waste away and die once they had been bitten by the tsetse fly. South African settlers in Zululand had their cattle herds decimated by *nagana*, "the wasting disease." Game hunters had to traverse the hinterland on foot as the "fly disease" killed their transport animals. Settlers throughout sub-Saharan Africa were threatened with economic ruin as their labor force and their livestock became drowsy and inert, fell asleep, and then died.

All of the European powers were struck by the "colonial disease." British South Africa, the Belgian Congo, German West Africa, and the French sub-Saharan colonies, along with those territories still retained by Portugal, saw populations of natives and settlers alike almost destroyed by sleeping sickness. Between 1896 and 1906 in British-occupied Uganda 250,000 Africans perished. In the Congo basin at least half a million people were wiped out. Native animals such as waterbuck and antelopes were not affected, even though they carried the sickness, having built up a resistance over millions of years. It seems that the Europeans were partly responsible for these horrendous outbreaks. Originally confined to coastal belts, the large expeditions into the interior spread the disease into native kingdoms that had never encountered this devastating infection. Adding to the dispersal were large caravans of Arab slave

BELOW **Officials question Ugandan locals in 1913 while serving on a commission set up to tackle the disease.**

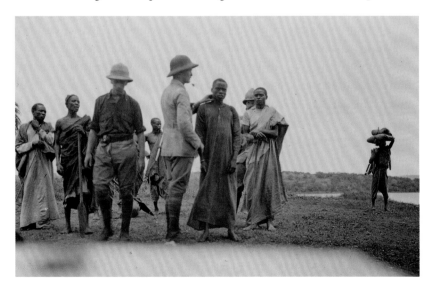

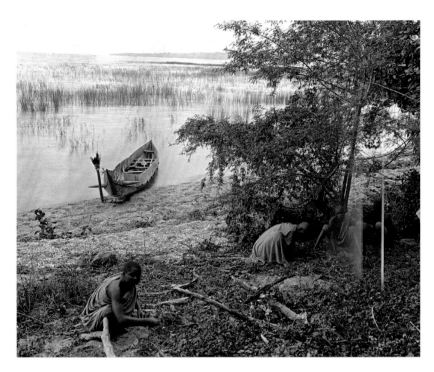

ABOVE **The same commissioners (see caption, page 179) took this photograph. It shows sufferers struggling to stay active in the throes of the disease.**

traders, who moved huge numbers of captives from infected areas in Central Africa to the northwest of Africa. Epidemics have persisted into recent times and the last major outbreak was in the 1970s, although in some regions it lasted into the 1990s.

There are three types of trypanosomiasis, all with different ranges and hosts, but all are devilishly clever in their ability to outwit and overcome human defenses. They are nearly impossible to wipe out as they live in many animals and humans throughout Africa and these multiple hosts facilitate breakouts at any time. Trypanosomes are covered with proteins to protect them from human defense mechanisms such as white blood cells. The host's immune system recognizes the protein and produces different antibodies, which then act to destroy the parasites as they circulate around the blood. But the trypanosomes are prepared for this assault and a small number will morph their protective coats into a new protein that is not recognized by the host's antibodies. This can happen several times until the immune system loses this microscopic arms race and is overwhelmed by the invading parasites. This is only part of the parasite's deadly armory; they multiply by "binary fission." This is where the creature replicates by splitting down the middle, doubling its numbers every few hours without any need for a more prolonged sexual reproductive process. In addition, the tryptophol chemical compound that induces sleep in humans is produced by the trypanosome parasite in sleeping sickness.

The seemingly harmless-looking trypanosomes, small thread-like worms with bulbous heads and spiral tails, are injected by the tsetse fly under the skin into the subcutaneous tissue. The tsetse bites are very painful and impossible to ignore, and two to three weeks after a bite, symptoms begin to develop. The trypanosomes breed in a person's fat before migrating to the bloodstream and lymphatic system. This first stage is the "hemolymphatic" stage where the bug gets a hold on the victim's system. An outward sign of this stage is "Winterbottom's sign," a large bubo-like swelling located on a lymph node in the neck, underarm, or groin. These painful pustule-like growths sometimes appear in the mouth, nose, or even eyeball, leading to excruciating pain and an inability to function properly. Often the tsetse fly bites refuse to heal, leading to painful sores or chancres. As well as these outward symptoms, the infected experience bouts of fever, headaches, joint pains, and itchy skin rashes. The kidneys and heart can also deteriorate.

In the second stage things get really serious. The parasites cross the blood–brain barrier and cause the neurological or meningoencephalitic phase of the assault. The nasty little brutes begin to effectively dissolve the host's central nervous system. The victim becomes confused, irritable, delusional, and unable to perform simple tasks due to lack of coordination. The invaders also infiltrate the brain, leading to irregular and disturbed sleep patterns with victims waking at all hours of the night and unable to go back to sleep, and then becoming drowsy and lethargic during the day. Personality changes are seen, while slurred speech, seizures, and difficulty in talking become evident, as well as extreme fatigue combined with aching muscles and joints. Eventually eating and basic functions become impossible and, several months or years after the initial symptoms, death is the inevitable outcome. Without treatment, the disease is invariably fatal, with progressive mental deterioration leading to coma, systemic organ failure, and death. Damage caused in the neurological phase is irreversible. As well as the behavioral symptoms displayed in this last phase of the disease, many patients display a "moon face." This is when the facial features become swollen and pale with the rupturing of small blood vessels.

The condition has been present in Africa for thousands of years but, due to the tribal nature of African society before Muslim and European colonization, there was not much travel between indigenous people and sleeping sickness in humans was limited to small isolated pockets. In the 17th

BELOW **The tsetse fly carries one of the cruelest diseases known to man, African trypanosomiasis. A small bite leads to a host of painful symptoms.**

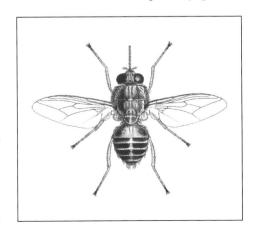

century this changed as Arab slave traders entered Central Africa from the east, following the Congo River, bringing parasites along with them. Originally known as "Gambian sleeping sickness," the disease traveled up the Congo River and then farther eastward.

The signs of sleeping sickness were easy to recognize and affected all races and classes. Arabs penetrated into the heart of Africa well before Europeans arrived. A Muslim visitor to the kingdom of Mali in the 14th century noticed that even the "sultan" of the kingdom was affected by the disease. In important meetings of state sleep was continually overtaking the man and it was impossible to wake him, making the transaction of official functions impracticable.

John Atkins (1685–1757), a British naval surgeon, described the disease and the devastating effect it had on slaves when he returned from West Africa:

> *The Sleepy Distemper (common among the Negroes) gives no other previous notice than a want of appetite 2 or 3 days before; their sleeps are sound, and sense and feeling very little; for pulling, drubbing or whipping will scarce stir up sense and power enough to move; and the moment you cease beating the smart is forgot, and down they fall again into a state of insensibility, driveling constantly from the Mouth as in deep salivation; breathe slowly, but not unequally nor snort. Young people are more subject to it than the old; and the Judgement generally pronounced is death, the prognostic seldom failing. If now and then one of them recovers, he certainly loses the little reason he had, and turns idiot...*
> —JOHN ATKINS, 1742

Identifying the Cause of Sleeping Sickness

Two case studies of colonial Europeans led to the identification of the cause of sleeping sickness. In May 1901 a 42-year-old steamer captain on the Gambia River in West Africa, Mr. Kelly, complained of feeling unwell with a slight fever. Consulting Dr. Robert Michael Forde, the Colonial Office's local surgeon, Kelly was initially diagnosed with malaria. However, the doctor could not identify any malaria parasites and the patient did not respond to quinine. Forde did observe some "wriggly worms" on blood slides and he noticed that their number ebbed and flowed in line with the intensity of Kelly's fever. Dr. Joseph Everett was able to recognize the worms as trypanosomes and correctly assumed they were a human version of the nagana disease found in cattle.

LEFT **Trypanosoma in a blood smear.
The parasites are covered by proteins that
ensure they are not attacked by white blood cells.**

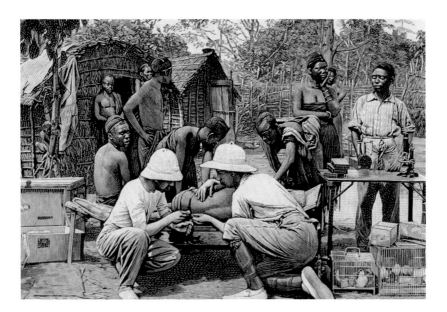

However, the diagnosis did not help Kelly, and he was sent home to England where he became more and more feverish before his heart failed in 1903. A Mrs. S., a missionary's wife returned from the Congo, was the second English case of sleeping sickness to attract the attention of medical experts. In 1902 she was struck by a fever, and in 1903 the symptoms became much worse as her nervous system was attacked. She died in 1903. Using the information gathered from these two patients it was proven that a bacterial agent was not to blame, but rather the trypanosome parasite. The understanding of the role the tsetse fly played in the cycle soon followed.

ABOVE By 1903 European explorers were able to examine blood smears of the native populations when looking for African trypanosomiasis.

Sleeping Sickness Today

Nevertheless, despite control programs throughout the early part of the 20th century, another epidemic of sleeping sickness broke out in the 1970s. Countries such as Uganda, The Democratic Republic of Congo, Sudan, The Central African Republic, and Angola saw millions of people die as civil wars, the refugee crisis, and economic decline caused health services to collapse and allowed the tsetse fly to return in plague proportions. Even today there are few effective medical treatments and up to 60,000 deaths occur each year. Pentamidine is an antimicrobial formula that, when administered intravenously, can knock out the infection if the diagnosis is made early enough.

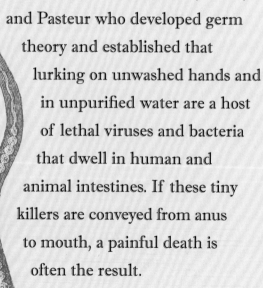

CHAPTER 9

ON FECAL MATTERS

As early as 1546 Girolamo Fracastoro, an Italian philosopher, surmised that epidemics were created by tiny "seeds" that were transmitted by direct contact. It was later scientists such as Semmelweiss, Snow, and Pasteur who developed germ theory and established that lurking on unwashed hands and in unpurified water are a host of lethal viruses and bacteria that dwell in human and animal intestines. If these tiny killers are conveyed from anus to mouth, a painful death is often the result.

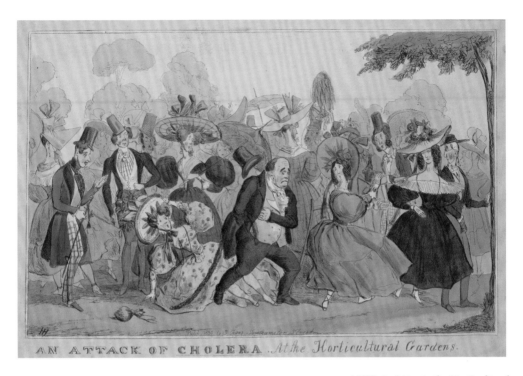

AN ATTACK OF CHOLERA. *At the Horticultural Gardens.*

CHOLERA

Initially emerging from Asia, cholera was, and is, a particularly nasty disease. A water-borne bacterium, it struck young and old, wealthy and poor. As a classic crowd disease, cholera was able to propagate and thrive in urban areas due to the huge amount of diarrhea that was expelled as the victim expired. It was greatly feared, not only because it killed nine out of ten of those infected, but because it struck seemingly at random and could kill in as little as three hours. The bacillus ate away at the lining of the intestine and a victim could void up to 3 gallons (12 liters) a day of watery diarrhea that contained small white flecks like ground rice.

ABOVE **A visitor to the Horticultural Society of London's gardens in Chiswick rushes off, believing he has cholera. This lethal disease could turn a healthy man into a wasted skeleton in hours.**

Cholera is caused by the bacterium *Vibrio cholerae*, which originated in the Ganges Delta in India and first broke onto the world stage in the 1800s. Once ingested, the bacteria multiply in the intestines (100 million bacteria are required to set off an infection) and release toxins, breaking down the lining of the gut and giving the expelled waste its characteristic rice-water appearance. About 75 percent of people infected with *V. cholerae* do not develop any symptoms, although the bacteria are present in their feces for 7 to 14 days after infection and are shed back into the environment, potentially infecting other people. Among people who develop symptoms,

185

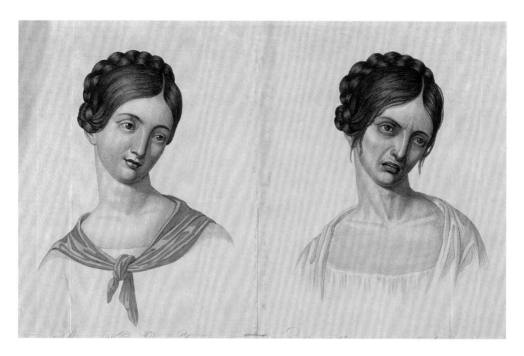

ABOVE **The horrors of cholera. This beautiful Viennese woman turns blue as a lack of fluids prevents oxygen getting to the skin.**

around 80 percent have mild or moderate symptoms, while the remainder develop acute watery diarrhea with severe dehydration. This can lead to death if untreated. People with low immunity—such as malnourished children or people living with HIV—are at a greater risk of death if infected.

The usual symptoms of cholera are profuse diarrhea and vomiting. An almost clear fluid is discharged and these symptoms usually start suddenly between 12 and 100 hours after ingesting the bacteria. The diarrhea is frequently compared to rice water and may have a fishy odor. The word "cholera" comes from the Greek for "bile" and this is another characteristic appearance. An untreated person with cholera may produce two to three gallons (10 to 20 liters) of diarrhea a day. Another possible Greek origin of the word is the term for a roof gutter, giving a vivid description of the fecal matter pouring out of the anus like rain out of a gutter during a downpour. The cholera bacteria produce and secrete toxins that trick the cells of the intestines into expelling prodigious quantities of water. Severe cholera, without treatment, kills about half of affected individuals. If the severe diarrhea is not treated, it can result in life-threatening dehydration and electrolyte imbalances. In extreme cases the person's skin turns blue, as lack of oxygen, due to poor circulation caused by lack of fluids, results in not enough oxygen getting to the skin. Other symptoms include sunken eyes and wrinkled hands or feet, as the extremities lose moisture. Blood pressure drops due to dehydration.

Scourge of the Ganges

Cholera had its origins in the Indian subcontinent and has been endemic to the Ganges River for hundreds and maybe thousands of years. Hot temperatures, pools of warm, stagnant still water, and large amounts of human and animal waste made this the perfect environment for the bacteria to enter the human population. *Vibrio cholerae* was named after its characteristic, vibrating wiggle. It only exists in humans but it has many water-borne relatives and it may have developed from a free-living *Vibrio* found in the Ganges before adapting to the human gut; or it may have transferred across the species divide when people ate infected fish or drank polluted water.

The first reference to a cholera-like disease was written in Sanskrit in the first millennium BCE. The writer described a disease that caused violent vomiting and diarrhea, muscle spasms, and a blue face. It remained in this region for thousands of years, probably adapting to water storage tanks. The development of new trade routes in the 19th century allowed the disease to become a worldwide phenomenon. Seemingly unstoppable pandemics erupted out of India and established the disease in thriving metropolises in Russia, Europe, America, Africa, and Asia. Seven pandemics have occurred in the last 200 hundred years, with the first originating in Bengal in 1817 and the last emerging from Indonesia in 1961.

The first cholera pandemic spread from Bengal and for the next seven years it raged through Southeast Asia, China, Japan, and the Middle East before it petered out around the Black Sea in southern Russia. In 1827 the previously untouched continents of Europe and North America were

BELOW **By the time of the 1893 epidemic in India, vaccinations were available to members of the British armed forces.**

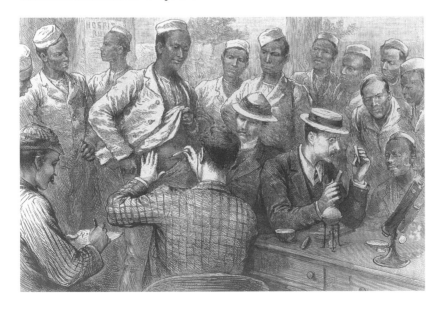

ravaged and technological advances helped propagate the disease as well as informing populations that the new killer disease was heading their way. Subsequent pandemics in 1839, 1863, 1881, and 1899 ensured that no inhabited part of the globe escaped the dreadful scourge.

The developments brought by colonial rule (roads, railroads, and busy ports) also benefited cholera, which erupted from an insignificant village somewhere outside Calcutta (Kolkata) in the first pandemic in 1817. Five thousand British soldiers were killed in the first weeks of the outbreak, which faded out after exacting a dreadful toll. It paused before Europe but in 1826 it resumed its deadly march and hit Afghanistan, Persia (Iran), and southern Russia. In 1830 it hit Moscow causing a mortality rate of over 50 percent. The city emptied as fleeing residents carried it to other Russian cities such as the capital, St. Petersburg. From there it reached Poland and Germany, before jumping ship to England. Irish migrants took it to Mexico, Cuba, and the United States.

The population was terrified of this strange new visitation. The first casualty in England was pretty 12-year-old Isabella Hazard. In October 1831 the lass had just attended church and was hale and healthy. She then felt a mild twinge of discomfort in her belly before she was overcome by stomach pains, vomiting, unquenchable thirst, spasms, and jet-like diarrhea of unimaginable force that drained her small body of liquid and caused her to turn blue. Her foul-smelling rice-water feces contained the bacteria as well as the lining of her gut. Such was the fluid loss that her blood could no longer circulate and she died, the first of 130,000 British victims. People could be fine in the morning and dead by teatime.

The epidemic of 1831 spread throughout Europe, although many states sought to limit its spread through quarantine. This was not successful and the disease swept through the continent, including Russia, seemingly targeting the poor in their low-standard, crowded accommodation. Quarantine, inefficient as it was, led to

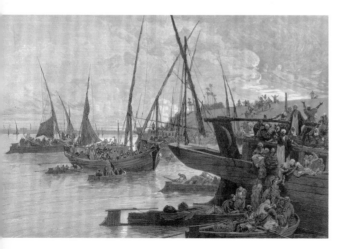

LEFT **Egyptians boarding boats on the Nile during a cholera epidemic. Cholera originated in India but spread through Europe and the Mediterranean.**

RIGHT **A depiction of cholera in** *Le Petit Journal.* **Cholera inspired fear as it wreaked its deadly toll throughout Europe. Wealth was no guarantee of safety.**

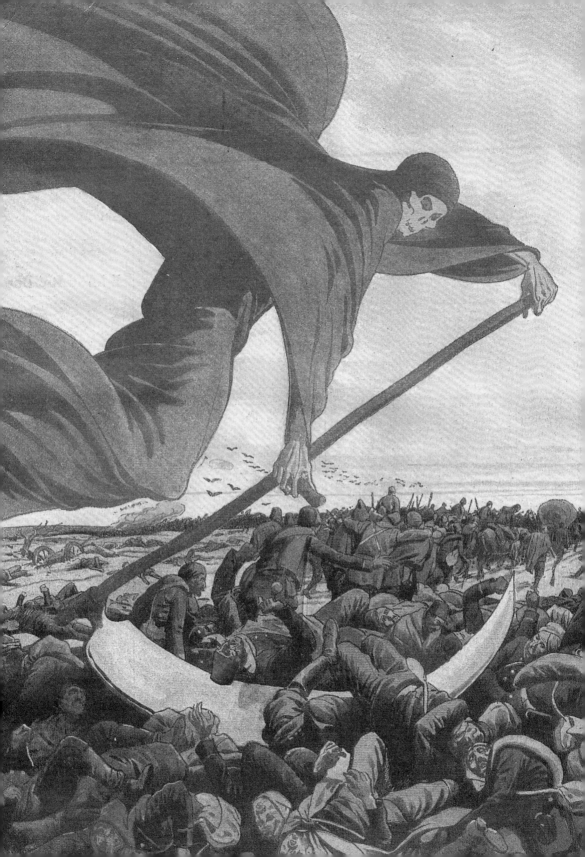

higher food prices, exacerbating the problems of society's disadvantaged. Riots broke out throughout Europe as hysteria took hold. Rumors spread that the disease was in fact a result of poisoning by the authorities who were trying to destroy any agents of possible rebellion. Peasants and doctors were massacred in Russia, as were policemen trying to cordon off infected sections of the population. In Hungary 100,000 died; surviving peasants turned on their superiors and sacked castles, killing the nobles. In Prussia it was rumored that doctors were paid a bounty for every peasant they infected, leading to public lynching and stoning of medical practitioners, occurrences that were mirrored in Paris. On the Indian subcontinent, where the disease originated, it was seen as deliberate poisoning of poor Indians by the colonial authorities.

Toward a Solution

In England inappropriate cures were sought to help the desperate victims hang on to life. Roast beef, bread, and potatoes were recommended as a preventative, and it was suggested that vegetables and fruit be excluded from the diet. Doses of brandy, sulfuric acid, laudanum, and ammonia were advocated for the sick, as well as placing hot bricks on their tortured bodies.

BELOW **This bizarre cholera safety suit of 1832 offered no protection from the deadly pathogen, which is transmitted via water.**

Even before the discovery of the cholera bacterium by the German bacteriologist Robert Koch in 1883, a link had been made between sewage and the disease. An appeal published in *The Times* in 1849 was a desperate plea for the British government to take notice:

Sir, we aint got no privis, no dust bins, no drains, no water supplies and no drain or suer in the hole place. The Suer company, in Greek Street, Soho Square, all great, rich powerfool men take no notice watsomdever of our complaints. The stench of a Gulley-hole is disgustin. We all of us suffer, and numbers are ill, and if the Cholera comes Lord help us.
—THE TIMES, JULY 5, 1849

Just as Isabella Hazard was one of the first recorded victims of cholera, it was another young girl—the baby daughter of Thomas and Sarah Lewis—whose death led to a means of stopping its deadly ravages. The summer of 1854 was unusually hot and the infant fell ill in her Soho home. She began pouring out green watery stools that emitted a pungent smell, overwhelming her distraught mother's attempts to deal with the soiled diapers. She gave them a cursory wash in a bucket of water before disposing of the noxious mix into a cesspool at the front of their rude tenement at 40 Broad Street. The following day,

AN INDUSTRIAL KILLER

CHOLERA WAS ABLE TO TAKE SUCH a hold on European cities at the time due to the effects of the Agricultural and Industrial Revolutions. Land clearance and the enclosure of common land had led to hundreds of thousands of agricultural tenants and leaseholders being kicked off the land and unable to practice farming for sustenance except during harvesting or sowing times.

And where did this growing population of dispossessed farm workers go? To the towns, where the Industrial Revolution was gaining pace. As new techniques revolutionized farming, so did the steam engine and spinning jenny transform both light and heavy manufacturing industries. These new industries required a compliant, centralized workforce and the rural folk migrating to the cities were perfect fodder for exploitation within the factory—and infection from new crowd diseases. The new class of urban poor had moved from their healthy, rural environment, where running water could be freely drawn and they lived in family units in individual houses, to an urban environment that must have seemed like a living hell to the recently arrived rural folk.

The reported deaths from cholera during the Industrial Revolution are

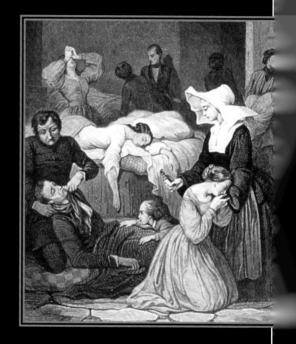

ABOVE In the crowded slums of Europe, infected waste ended up in privies. From there the infection spread to the water table, then to wells in a vicious cycle of reinfection.

mind-numbing. In 1831, 1848, and 1853 the numbers of deaths in London alone were respectively 6,536, 14,137, and 10,738. These epidemics were not confined to poor areas such as Soho or Bermondsey but also struck select, fashionable Mayfair. The final epidemic of 1866 struck only in Whitechapel, a notorious area of depravity and prostitution, where it killed at least 5,000 people.

cholera swept through the neighborhood and within ten days 10 percent of the local population, some 500 people, were dead.

A young, teetotal, vegetarian doctor, John Snow, investigated the outbreak and noted with meticulous detail where all the victims had obtained their water and food. The one common denominator was that they had all got their drinking water from one pump. This pump was located directly in front of 40 Broad Street. The pump was turned off and the cholera abated. At 40 Broad Street (now 39 Broadwick Street) there is now a pub, fittingly called "The John Snow."

Although it was not the end of cholera outbreaks, Snow's discovery was the first chink in the armor of the "miasmists" who believed cholera was transmitted through foul air. An example of the strength of the miasmists' beliefs is this quote from an 1847 report explaining the plethora of illnesses in the English capital:

> *This disease mist, arising from the breath of two millions of people, from open sewers and cesspools, graves and slaughter houses, is continually kept up and undergoing changes; in one season it is pervaded by Cholera; in another by Influenza; at one time it bears Smallpox, Measles, Scarlatina and Whooping Cough among your children; in another it carries fever on its wings. Like an angel of death it has hovered for centuries over London.*
> —*JOURNAL OF THE STATISTICAL SOCIETY OF LONDON*
> (VOLUME 10, NO. 3), SEPTEMBER 1847

Such sentiments were attractive to politicians as it meant they did not have to spend money on new infrastructure. But evidence such as Snow's and Koch's had established the connection between polluted water and a range of diseases, including cholera. Progressive improvements in sewage disposal and treatment over the latter half of the 19th century saw cholera almost disappear in industrialized countries.

LEFT **The Broad Street pump, Soho, London, was the epicenter of a cholera outbreak that killed 500 people in 1854. Physician John Snow linked the outbreak to water from this pump.**

Terrible Waste

During the European Industrial Revolution in the 18th and 19th centuries, profit was king, and without government regulations the urban poor became the fuel that was burned and sacrificed to satisfy the ever-growing demands of the mercantile classes. Crowded into filthy tenements built using shoddy materials, these town dwellers lacked even the most basic amenities. No sewerage system was in place, and human waste was stored in cesspits or washed down the center of the street in a providential rainfall. Privies were of the "long drop" variety and were known by various names such as the "gong house," the "place of easement," and the "bog house." Entire apartment blocks often had to share one, and the feces of up to 100 people would be deposited before the night-soil man could come and collect it, with a view to selling it on as fertilizer. However, demand for night soil never exceeded supply, and some of the poorest districts' privies were left unemptied and filled up before overflowing into basements or waterways. Even towns that were largely rural but had some industry—

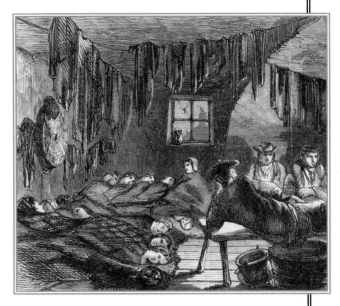

ABOVE **A wood engraving depicting the cramped and squalid housing conditions prevalent in tenements. Below the crowded tenements were privies, large holes filled with years of accumulated human waste.**

such as Haworth in Yorkshire, where the Brontë sisters were brought up—couldn't manage their waste, and thousands died on a regular basis.

The first modern toilets were designed by such luminaries as Thomas Crapper and had imaginative names such as "The Deluge," "Niagara Falls," and "Waterloo." Many of these early water closets were installed in the houses of the wealthy, but without a functioning sewerage system the waste from them still found its way back into the water table or local waterways.

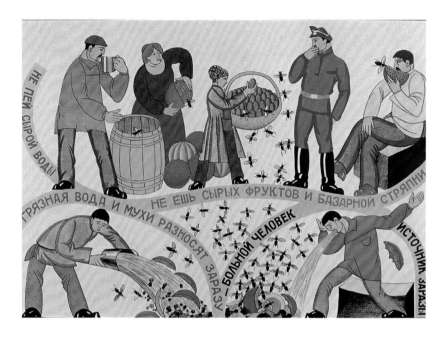

ABOVE **Soviet authorities recognized the dangers posed by cholera. This Ukrainian poster from the Kiev region in 1921 promotes proper hygiene.**

Cholera Today

Cholera is still a major killer in developing countries. In 1961 a new strain of *Vibrio cholerae* burst out of Indonesia. Named El Tor (after a city in Egypt), this strain was hardier and easier to transmit than any of its predecessors and caused a major pandemic that lasted for 30 years. It moved in repeated waves through Southeast Asia and hit 29 countries in Africa. It reached Peru in 1991 and raced like wildfire through the abominably poor inhabitants of the shantytowns of Lima. The population had soared in two decades from 1 million to 7 million and the city's waste networks were unable to cope with the increased population even when they were in good health. When up to 4,500 people a day were being struck down with the dreadful disease, hundreds of thousands of gallons of infected "rice water" feces overwhelmed the sewerage system every day. The tainted sewage penetrated the water supply, which the government had ceased to chlorinate. One hundred and fifty thousand cases were reported and in some regions the mortality rate exceeded 10 percent.

The outbreak originated from ballast flushed from ships arriving from Asia; it was communicated to the human population through the local tradition of eating ceviche, a dish made from raw fish.

During 1991, Colombia, Chile, Bolivia, Ecuador, Argentina, Brazil, and Guatemala all experienced outbreaks with a minimum of half a million being infected. Cholera remains a nasty and deadly disease.

Postmortem Photography

VICTORIANS ON BOTH SIDES of the Atlantic developed corpse preservation into an art form. Photographers became skilled at posing the dead to make them look lifelike using props and makeup. They were often posed with living family members to accentuate what they looked like in life. The saddest Victorian death photos are those that show entire families or sets of siblings laid low by an outbreak of disease. This practice of immortalizing the dead was known as memorial portraiture.

Supports and gadgets were used to make the body look as lifelike as possible. Corpses were posed using frames to support them to stand or sit, while some practitioners painted lifelike eyes on their closed eyelids. Young women were often dressed in wedding gowns to show what they would have looked like had they lived to see their own wedding day. Children were often portrayed with living siblings or with parents, or with favorite objects such as dolls or pets. Many were photographed as if peacefully sleeping, but the ravages of disease are often present in the hollow cheeks and sunken eyes of the dead, belying any attempt to make them appear alive. Sometimes makeup was applied or the photographic image tinted to give the victims rosy cheeks.

The fact that the photographer was able to arrange the cadaver in a lifelike pose indicates that the session took place at least 36 hours after death. Six to eight hours after death rigor mortis sets in, and 24 to 84 hours afterward the body becomes flaccid. However, it is impossible to get a dead hand to grasp a loved one's limbs, and eyes of the dead could not focus on an object, so they seem to gaze silently into space. Often the body must have emitted quite a stench, but such was the bond between members of a family that the love they held for their deceased relative shines through in these photos.

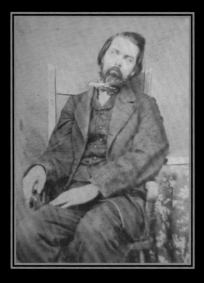

LEFT A skilled postmortem photographer could pose cadavers so that they looked alive. The slack hands were a dead giveaway, though.

Typhoid Fever

Typhoid is an unpleasant disease that follows a common transmission route, the fecal–oral route. Infected carriers who do not wash their hands properly after going to the toilet transmit the bacterium *Salmonella typhi*. It can also be found in infected water, and spreads rapidly in areas of poor sanitation and inadequate hygiene. Typhoid is probably an heirloom disease, or has been around in the human ecosystem for a long time, as it is not as lethal as many other pathogens.

Typhoid has a fatality rate of 10 to 20 percent if untreated. It causes a range of symptoms including abdominal pain, blinding headache, a rash, and a high fever. A few days after exposure, the patient experiences a splitting headache, chills, and loss of appetite. The body temperature then rises to 104 or 105° Fahrenheit (40 to 40.5° Celsius), and remains high for up to two weeks. A characteristic rash appears on the abdomen, followed by severe cramping in the guts, diarrhea, and general soreness. Historically, cold baths or wet towels were often applied to bring down the temperature. The disease usually lasted for about a month and lowered resistance to other infections. Patients who were already ill were the most likely to die.

BELOW **This illustration displays how typhoid bacteria were able to migrate between sewerage networks and water sources.**

One of the earliest incidences of typhoid in the historical record may be the death of Alexander the Great (323 BCE).

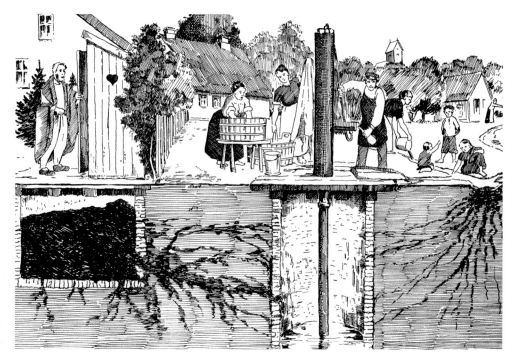

An Urban Disease

Typhoid was very much an urban disease. Victorian London was hit hard by an outbreak whenever the Thames flooded, pushing feces into the fresh water supplies. Prince Albert, the beloved husband of Queen Victoria, was one of the most celebrated victims. In 1861 he drank contaminated water and came down with typhoid. He had a high fever, was covered in violent rose-colored spots (one of the reasons typhoid was often confused with typhus), and vomited repeatedly. The best physicians money could buy were in attendance and diagnosed "bowel fever," but little could be done and on December 14, 1861, the 41-year-old prince died. Queen Victoria fell into a grief-filled stupor and never fully recovered from her loss.

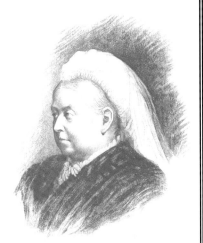

ABOVE **Queen Victoria lost the love of her life, Prince Albert, to typhoid fever in 1861. She became dour and reserved after this tragedy.**

Theories abound as to the cause of his death, malaria or poison being likely culprits. Research published in the *New England Journal of Medicine* in 1998 reported that the symptoms of the dying 32-year-old ruler were possibly related to typhoid. They included chills, exhaustion, sweats, severe abdominal pain, and a high fever. Though of course there is no proof, we do know that he died in Babylon, where urban sewage is likely to have contaminated the Euphrates River, the main source of drinking water.

A later historical outbreak of typhoid occurred when the original English settlers founded Jamestown in Virginia in the early 17th century. They did so near the banks of the James River, which encircled the tiny settlement on three sides. Not only was the site easily defendable, but also they thought that the river would wash away their waste material. Unfortunately they were wrong, and as they shed germs in their feces into the water, the current was too weak, particularly in summer, to wash it away. Possibly 6,000 of the early settlers were killed by typhoid between 1607 and 1624. Many were well aware of the pestilential nature of the water. George Percie, one of the original settlers, wrote: "Our drink, cold water taken out of the river, which was at a flooded state, very salty, and at low tide, full of slime and filth, was the destruction for many of our men."

A Human Disease

The typhoid bacillus was identified in the early 1880s. Typhoid has its own unique identity and life cycle. In 1896, the Widal test was developed to identify the bacterium, named after Georges-Fernand Widal who introduced it. It was realized that the only carrier for typhoid was man, and once methods for cleaning water supplies were adopted, such as those used to stop cholera outbreaks, it was only necessary to control human hosts from infecting others.

So effective were the controls on water supplies that typhoid was eliminated as a pathogen in the drinking water from many major cities in the West. Typhoid does not always show up as a full-blown infection in many people. Often the disease will infect a person but only produce mild symptoms such as a sniffle or a short-lived fever. The infected person can nevertheless shed bacteria. These bacteria pass down the bile duct with the bile and enter the intestines, where they mix with undigested food and ultimately feces and urine before being excreted. Thus, the stools of the carriers are heavily infected and the bacteria live on in the pancreas of infected persons. The typhoid bacteria breed within the gallbladder without any apparent harm to the host. Routinely, bacteria increase their numbers and move into the gut before they are expelled along with feces. Thus harmless-appearing carriers can move among their fellow human beings without any indication that they harbor a lethal pathogen. Most do not infect others, but some who work in the food industry and do not clean their hands after going to the toilet can infect many people.

Typhoid Mary

The most famed carrier who infected many innocent people was Mary Mallon (1869–1938), known as "Typhoid Mary." Mary Mallon was a cook who was well appreciated by the wealthy households who employed her. One of the most popular dishes that she prepared was freshly peeled peaches on vanilla ice cream. The problem was that as Mary peeled and sliced the delicious fresh peaches, the juice ran under her fingernails and dislodged some feces that had lodged there last time she used the "facilities." Mary didn't believe in washing her hands and as she placed the peach slices on top of the ice cream, minute samples of fecal matter that were infected with *Salmonella typhi* were added to the dish. As her appreciative clients wolfed down the

LEFT **Mary Mallon was an excellent cook and a model employee except for one fact: she did not wash her hands after using the toilet.**

delicious confection, little did they know that six of the eleven family members would be struck down with the life-threatening disease, typhoid.

Mary first came to the attention of the authorities when the family of wealthy investment banker Charles Henry Warren was struck down with typhus while they were renting a luxurious holiday house in Oyster Bay, Long Island. In 1906, six members of the Warren household were ill and George Thompson, the owner of the house, hired a private investigator to determine the source of the outbreak. George Soper was given the task of tracking down the vector, as Thompson wanted to be able to prove that the infection was not within the structure of the house, to ensure he could re-let it. As medical knowledge of bacterial infections grew, so too grew an industry dedicated to tracking it down and eliminating possible sources. Some of this effort came from the public purse while individuals too paid to ensure the safety of their family or their tenants.

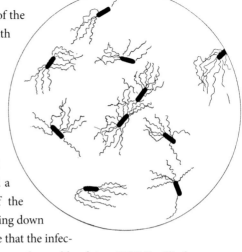

ABOVE **Bacilli of typhoid fever, grown in a culture.**

Soper was a civil engineer who was seen as something of a typhoid fever epidemic specialist. He began by interviewing the Warren family. The first to fall ill had been one of Warren's daughters, followed by two maids, Mrs. Warren, another daughter, and then the gardener. Soper examined and eliminated all possible vectors such as preserved foods, water, local clams, and any suspect outsiders. The one clue that paid off was that the family had hired a new cook two weeks before the outbreak in August 1906: Mary Mallon.

Displaying how investigations of this nature had become commonplace by the early 20th century, Soper was able to use his expertise to establish Mallon's employment history since 1897. A disturbing pattern emerged, showing that in each place she had worked, people were struck down with typhoid.

Soper determined to prove his theory by collecting fecal matter, urine, and blood from Mallon. Her feces produced overwhelming amounts of typhoid bacilli when they were tested at the Willard Packer Hospital in New York. In 1902 the German bacteriologist Robert Koch had suggested that convalescing patients could shed typhoid bacteria in their feces even after they had recovered their health. The question that Koch could not answer was how long the patients would continue to shed the bacteria in their feces. Mary Mallon solved that question: as much as 30 percent of the bacteria discovered in her stool and urine samples was *Salmonella typhi*.

Such was the potential danger of such a carrier that Mary was moved to an isolation cottage on the grounds of the Riverside Hospital on North Brother Island in

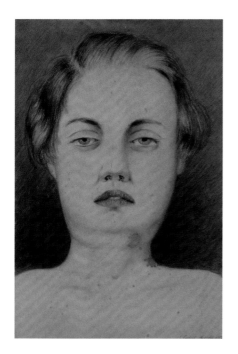

ABOVE **A patient in the throes of typhoid fever. A bloody nose and rash accompanying a high fever are characteristic of the disease.**

New York. She was kept in this facility for two years until she managed to obtain her release. In the 28 months between March 1907 and June 1909 her feces were tested 163 times. She was what was categorized as an intermittent carrier. At one stage no bacilli were detected over 12 consecutive tests; however, 120 of the 163 cultures did test positive. Her urine was always clear. Mallon was determined to be released and sponsored her own tests. Although these showed no signs of typhoid, the New York City Health Department relied on its own findings and kept her incarcerated.

Mary refused to acknowledge her responsibility for causing outbreaks and that is why she was not released. Only when she signed a deposition swearing to avoid any job that involved food handling were the city authorities willing to let her go. She was soon employed as a laundress but, finding the pay and conditions not to her liking, she obtained work as the hospital cook in Sloane Maternity Hospital in Manhattan. Twenty-four people were infected and two died. An investigation revealed that the cook, a Mrs. Brown, was in fact Mary Mallon and she was again hauled off to North Brother Island. She remained there until her death in 1938 and this was no doubt an appropriate punishment since she had knowingly or unknowingly caused the deaths of two innocent people. During this time she continued to provide stool samples, often against her will, and they showed recurrent typhoid until she died.

Chronic Carriers

Medical practice at the turn of the 20th century labeled people with Mary's condition as "healthy carriers," "chronic carriers," or "germ distributors." While most modern nations in the late 19th and early 20th centuries upgraded their water systems by a process of filtration and separation from contaminated sources, there was still a large residual human population that carried the bug and it was the responsibility of health departments to identify these carriers. It was believed that the bacilli resided in the gallbladder and many of those who were thought to pose a risk were encouraged to have this organ removed. Usually the suspects were tracked down, tested, and asked not to be involved in jobs that required food preparation. Investigations revealed that approximately 3 percent of those who survived typhoid fever went on to be chronic carriers. Middle-aged women had a higher percentage in this category.

The numbers could be staggering. In 1910 there were 200,000 cases of reported typhoid in the United States, of whom at least 6,000 were likely to become "germ distributors" and pose a real threat to those surrounding them. Authorities carried out bacterial research just as Soper did to track down Mallon. In 1909 an outbreak in the Bronx was caused by a dairyman who harbored the bacilli, and infected milk as it was being processed for distribution. He was forced out of his job but, unlike Mary, acquiesced to the demand to leave his career and so was not confined in quarantine. Sweeps were also conducted where the stools of all registered food handlers were inspected, although the magnitude of this task made it a somewhat doubtful proposition. In the years following these outbreaks a name-and-shame list was produced which identified 70 high-risk carriers who were closely monitored. Three were confined (including Mary) and several were pretty much kept in house arrest.

As the carriers from earlier outbreaks died out and water quality improved, typhoid fever became rare in Western countries. Moreover, a vaccine was developed by World War I, and an effective drug was developed, which was first marketed in 1948 under the name "chloramphenicol." Nevertheless, it is still a scourge of developing countries and worldwide there are approximately 17 million cases per year resulting in at least 60,000 deaths. Adding to concerns is the fact that, like tuberculosis, some strains of *Salmonella typhi* are becoming resistant to many antibiotics.

BELOW African-American flood refugees are vaccinated for typhoid at Camp Louisiana near Vicksburg in the 1930s.

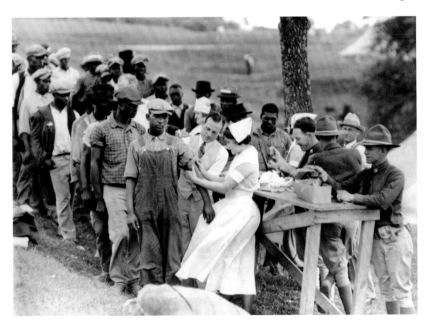

DYSENTERY

Dysentery is easily treatable today but in the past, with poor hygiene, it could be life-threatening. There are two kinds of dysentery. One, caused by the bacterium *Shigella*, is known as "bacillary dysentery." The other is amoebic dysentery, caused by amoeba. The amoeba group together and form a cyst, and the cysts come out of the body in human feces. In areas of poor sanitation, these cysts (which can survive for a long time) can contaminate food and water and infect other humans. The cysts can also linger on infected people's hands after going to the toilet. Good hygiene practice reduces the risk of infecting other people. Shigellosis was, and is, the most common form, and even today 120 million cases occur worldwide. It commonly affects children in the developing world and there are at least 1.1 million deaths every year.

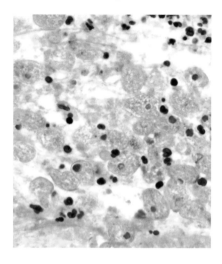

ABOVE **Histopathologic image of amoebic dysentery. The disease causes small cysts, easily identifiable in a colonic biopsy.**

Dysentery is an intestinal inflammation, especially in the colon, which can lead to severe diarrhea with mucus or blood in the feces. Sufferers typically experience mild to severe abdominal pain or stomach cramps. In some cases, untreated dysentery can be life-threatening, especially if the infected person cannot replace lost fluids fast enough. Those with a mild case may just have a runny, frequent stool (diarrhea) and slight stomach ache. Symptoms usually appear one to two days after infection. Severe dysentery can be a lot worse. Severe abdominal pain is accompanied by fever and chills, nausea and vomiting, and watery diarrhea that contains mucus and pus, followed by fatigue and dehydration. In these extreme cases, dysentery patients may pass more than two pints (one liter) of fluid per hour. Rectal pain, rapid weight loss, and generalized muscle soreness also accompany dysentery. On rare occasions, the amoebic parasite will invade the body through the bloodstream and spread beyond the intestines to infect other organs such as the brain, lungs, and liver.

DYSENTERY IS AN INTESTINAL INFLAMMATION, ESPECIALLY IN THE COLON, WHICH CAN LEAD TO SEVERE DIARRHEA WITH MUCUS OR BLOOD IN THE FECES. SUFFERERS TYPICALLY EXPERIENCE MILD TO SEVERE ABDOMINAL PAIN OR STOMACH CRAMPS.

The Bloody Flux

While not as deadly as typhoid or cholera, dysentery has made its mark on history. In 1216 King John of England died at Newark Castle and in 1422 Henry V died suddenly at the age of 35. Sir Francis Drake perished in 1596 while attacking Puerto Rico and in 1605 the Mughal emperor Akbar the Great perished from dysentery. The "bloody flux" killed many on campaign and contributed to the French death toll in Russia in 1812, and it is estimated to have killed 600,000 during the American Civil War in the years up until 1865.

In World War II this disease ravaged the concentration camp populations and was used by both the Russians and the Japanese as a means of controlling and humiliating prisoners.

On July 17, 1944, during the Soviet Union's Operation Bagration, 60,000 German soldiers were captured, the most grievous loss to the Wehrmacht of World War II. The prisoners were marched through the streets of Moscow. Many reasons were given for this march, including the need to prove to the disbelieving Western allies the scale of the Soviet triumph, as well as to give a morale boost to the tired Russian population. However, the main reason was to humiliate the German soldiers. Before the march they were given contaminated food and water, and as they paraded on Red Square, headed by 21 captured generals, diarrhea flooded down their legs, caused by dysentery. The stinking column of humiliated Germans were abused and pelted with missiles before being shipped to POW camps where 80 percent perished.

The Japanese capitalized on the unpleasantness of dysentery to force prisoners held in the Selarang Barracks of Changi Prison (Singapore) to sign a pledge not to seek to escape. The prisoners were not allowed to use the latrines and had to parade standing in their own waste for hours at a time until they did as the Japanese bid. Japanese ideology held that a healthy mind equated with a healthy body. While this could be attained on a reasonable diet, Allied prisoners of war were held in foul conditions for such an extended period of time that thousands died of a whole host of illnesses; but dysentery was the chief cause of mortality, causing up to 99 percent of deaths in some camps.

The camps rarely had running water, and basic needs of hygiene such as soap, toothpaste, and toilet paper were rarely supplied to the inmates. Watery douches with old rags were the most effective form of ablutions that most prisoners could expect, but some prisoners, such as the Dutch, had a reputation for using a bottle of water and their fingers. Others would use anything that came to hand if no toilet paper was issued, such as corncobs, bamboo, grass, and leaves. But all prisoners avoided the Japanese paper, which was rough like sandpaper. Toilets were usually long poles suspended over trenches, which would rapidly fill and often overflow in monsoon conditions. Flies, of course, flocked to these sites before plaguing the living quarters of the prisoners. They settled on men's faces while sleeping or dive-bombed their meager rice rations, flying into open mouths where they banged against the tongue and cheeks as they tried to escape. In these circumstances, most prisoners contracted dysentery during at least one part of their imprisonment.

Not only prisoners but also fighting soldiers throughout the Pacific often suffered from dysentery. Australian soldiers marching on the Kokoda track simply cut a hole in the rear of their trousers so they could march and fight without having to take time out and squat. Those suffering from dysentery were unpopular with their hut mates, as they would make a dash for the privies at all hours of the night, stamping on their sleeping fellows as they desperately raced for the long drop.

Many soldiers couldn't get to the toilets because they were also suffering from beriberi and malaria. Beriberi caused fluid buildups in the belly and testicles, making them swell to huge proportions while the patient's arms and legs became weak and spindly. This was caused by a lack of vitamin B1 and was common throughout Asia where the basic diet was rice-based. As for malaria, few Japanese camps issued their prisoners with quinine. Doctors would often see soldiers dashing for the latrine only to collapse as fever struck them, or as their emaciated legs were unable to take their weight. Beriberi caused edema (swelling) to such an extent that lungs filled up with fluids and the chest became so engorged that no neck could be seen until the patient was forced to take gulps of air like a frog croaking. Many died as their lungs were overwhelmed.

These poor conditions were largely due to neglect, which became worse when the Japanese supply lines were cut as the war progressed. However, in the Selarang Barracks incident thousands of POWs were forced to stand in their own feces for days as latrine pits overflowed and fresh water was cut off. Following the British surrender of Singapore on February 15, 1942, Allied POWs were ordered by the Japanese to march to Changi for internment. As the British-built Changi Prison was already crowded with Allied POWs and civilians, the surrounding barracks including Selarang were used by the Japanese as a holding area for Australian and British prisoners.

Under the Geneva Convention POWs were not to be punished if they sought to escape from a prisoner of war "cage." However, most of the men held in Selarang Barracks were still fighting fit, having after only spent a short time in captivity, and it was obvious to their captors that escape attempts would be made. The filth that would soon overwhelm the camp made this even more likely.

The Selarang Barracks was certainly not a place anybody would want to spend time in. It was originally built to house 800 men. It consisted of a parade ground the size of a football oval surrounded on three sides with barracks. As many as 17,000 men were forced to exist in this confined space, suffering under the tropical sun.

An Australian POW named George Aspinall was horrified by the situation. He noted that in each overcrowded barracks there were four to six toilets which were flushed with water from small cisterns on the barracks roof. The Japanese added to the torments of their prisoners by cutting the water off, making the toilets unusable. In the entire compound only one tap was made available and prisoners had to line up all day for the opportunity for a quick wash. One bottle of water was provided to each man per day, and this was used for both drinking and washing. Soon their rank waste overflowed onto the parade square, making it impossible to sit or relax.

The Japanese used several methods to try to prevent escapes. On August 30, 1942, the commander, General Shimpei Fukuye, tried to get the British and Australian soldiers to sign a "no escape pledge." This read in part: "I the undersigned, hereby solemnly swear on my honor that I will not, under any circumstances, attempt to escape." The prisoners, of course, refused to sign the document, with the exception of three men. They were not yet fully aware of the brutal methods the Japanese would use to enforce compliance.

Four prisoners who had attempted to escape some weeks earlier were executed by the Japanese in front of the Allied officers in charge of the POWs. The executions by sword were botched and all four men, three British and one Australian, had to be finished off with a pistol shot to the head. Despite the executions, or perhaps because of them, the prisoners resolve not to sign the documents remained firm. The Japanese were not deterred. They kicked the prisoners out of the barracks onto the square. Food and water were further limited and dysentery raged throughout the prison. Men condemned to stay outdoors in the tropical heat, covered in filth and without access to fluids soon began to die as dysentery became a lethal contagion.

BELOW **A young man suffering from dysentery. Most can survive a bout of dysentery. However, for those with weakened immune systems it can be fatal.**

The decision was made by the prisoners to sign the pledges. This was under duress, but the British and Australian commanders thought that their men's welfare made it necessary. However, as the men lined up to sign, they managed to pull the wool over their captors' eyes. The Japanese had little or no English and many Ned Kellys and Winston Churchills pledged not to escape. The Japanese allowed some measures of hygiene to be restored after the signing.

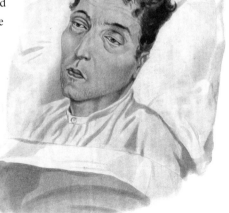

WORMS

Feces may also carry worm infestations. The most common forms are roundworms, which typically live in the human gut and, as their name suggests, have a round body. About 60 species of roundworms are parasites of humans. Cadavers from ancient times often have roundworm eggs preserved in their guts. Bog People from Northern Europe, such as Lindow Man found in an English peat swamp, were infested by a variety of gut bugs.

Buried with Lindow man, who was interned in a bog in approximately 50 CE, was evidence of parasitic infection. After his discovery in 1984, scientific research indicated that he was infested with two types of worms and their eggs were found in what remained of his digestive tract. Whipworm is one of the most common infectious worms found today and it has also turned up in other bog bodies as well as in privies from medieval times and from the Dark Ages. Following the usual course of most of these worm infections, whipworm (*Trichuris trichiura*) is taken into the body when fecal matter is transferred to the digestive system through unwashed hands, or where human waste is used to fertilize fields. The whipworm is a small, thin worm and lives in the large bowel. There are few symptoms for a mild infection of only a few worms, but if they are allowed to multiply beyond all control, symptoms can include poor appetite, feelings of weakness, weight loss, tiredness, abdominal pain, and diarrhea. There can be blood

BELOW **This section of intestine, removed from a three-year-old boy, displays how an unchecked worm infestation can prevent the host from absorbing nutrients.**

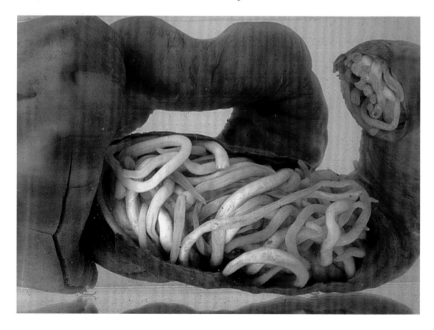

in the stool and if children are heavily infested they may have retarded development intellectually and physically, as well as anemia. Once established, the whipworm is hard to get rid of; a mature female can live for five years and produce 20,000 eggs a day.

Lindow man was also colonized by an even more unpleasant beast, the mawworm (*Ascaris lumbricoides*). This nasty creature is much larger than the whipworm, with the female growing up to 20 inches (50 cm) long with a width of less than ¼ inch (6 mm). The life cycle of this animal is particularly unpleasant. The fertilized eggs are ingested along with fecal matter and when in the small intestine they hatch into a larval worm that penetrates the gut wall and moves into the bloodstream. They are then carried to the liver and heart before migrating to the lungs where they break into the alveoli. There they grow and after three weeks they molt and irritate the lungs so that they are coughed up and swallowed to return to the small intestine where they mature into adult male or female worms. At this stage the worms breed. The female can produce up to 200,000 eggs per day for a year. These eggs can live for up to 10 years in soil.

Lindow man and his contemporaries may have tried herbal remedies to shift this menace, but the eggs have a tough outer layer that is resistant to acids and alkalis found in plant matter, making them, even today, hard to shift. The mawworm seems to have originated in pigs and seemingly crossed the species barrier many thousands of years ago. It can be deadly. Populations can migrate into the appendix, pancreas, kidneys, and brain where they burrow into their host using their three-toothed mouthpiece and cause catastrophic organ failure. They can also multiply in the intestines in such numbers that these organs are entirely blocked by the struggling, writhing mass. Urban legends talk of worms emerging from the rectum, mouth, and nose of deceased or starving hosts, and this does in fact happen. If no food is to be found in the lower intestine, this and other types of roundworms will seek to migrate out of the body in search of sustenance.

The Renaissance seems to have been an era when intestinal worms were particularly virulent. Accounts of the time speak of individuals wasted by parasitical invasions, and others suffering so much pain in their gut that they collapsed and violently convulsed while unconscious. A five-year-old child was found dead after worms had gnawed their way through his belly; and in the summer of 1655 an innkeeper allegedly voided an assortment of long worms with heads resembling a hound, a horse, and a toad!

Physician William Ramsey wrote in 1668 that even infants less than 12 months old could harbor so many parasites that they died of emaciation. He observed one fellow extruding a flatworm 7 feet (2 meters) long, and another patient had a grossly distended groin that split to reveal three huge, writhing worms. He witnessed other victims expelling "serpents" through their anuses, mouths, ears, and even penises.

10

MENTAL ILLNESS

WHILE MODERN TECHNOLOGY AND
knowledge allows us to diagnose and,
hopefully, treat this plethora of disorders,
earlier societies were much more likely
to blame supernatural forces for mental
illness, and punish or torture the sufferers.
Even as modern medical practices were
introduced and the "science" of mental
illness developed, cures were often
a lot worse than the maladies.

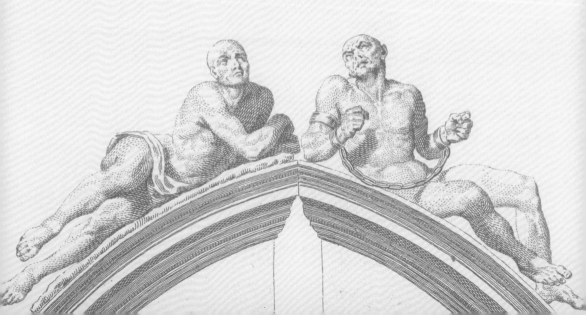

TOUCHED BY THE GODS

Ancient peoples had many ways of curing the mentally ill. In many primitive societies, the insane were seen as being touched by the gods. They could be elevated to shaman status, or else concoctions made from berries and barks would be administered by healers, or druids, to try to cure sufferers.

The classical Greek and Roman societies (500 BCE to 400 CE) used a variety of treatments. Opium could be administered along with cold baths, purges, trepanning (cutting a hole in the skull to let evil spirits out), and even electroshock therapy with electric eels. If live eels were not available, powdered eels would be mixed with olive oil and administered as a draft.

The ancient Greeks thought that madness was a punishment sent by the gods. Plato was the first to identify political protest with madness and propose a "house of sanity" to lock dissidents away. Epileptics or those displaying delusional symptoms were told to avoid baths, rich foods, and the wearing of black clothes. Greeks also believed that these disorders could be avoided if they did not wear goatskin, or cover one hand with the other. The Spartans killed any youths displaying abnormal tendencies.

BELOW **Doctors were respected in ancient Greek society and made many early diagnoses of mental illnesses.**

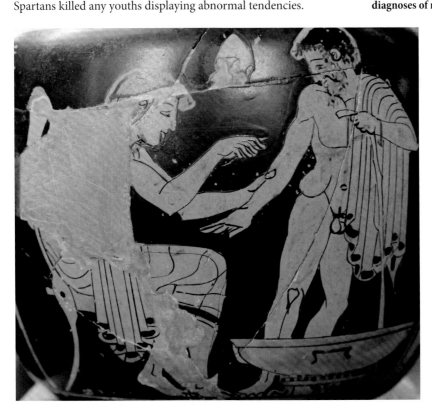

MISDIAGNOSED

In the past, a variety of mental illnesses would be diagnosed simply as bad humors. However, modern psychology recognizes a multiplicity of diseases that disrupt the mental health of millions. These include:

• Schizophrenia: Typically associated with hearing voices and accompanied by hallucinations and paranoid delusions.

• Somatization disorder: This used to be classed as hysteria and often psycho-somatic pains are associated with this. These can include nausea, depression, headaches, and paralysis.

• Bipolar disease: The patient alternates between periods of depression and periods of manic activity with verbose ideas of grandiosity.

• Depression: This used to be classified as melancholia and results in individuals retreating from society and having suicidal thoughts.

• Obsessive-compulsive disorder (OCD): Intrusive thoughts and anxieties lead to compulsive and repetitive behaviors.

• Tourette's syndrome: This creates uncontrollable tics and speech that is often abusive.

• Disassociation: An individual may feel unconnected with their body or not able to stop certain actions.

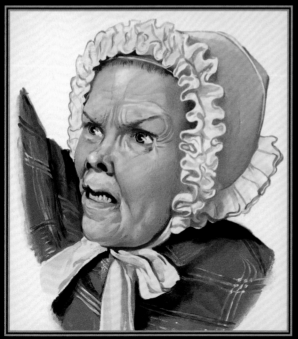

LEFT A woman diagnosed as suffering from "mania." This catch-all term could be applied to anyone suffering from mental instability.

The biblical Jews believed that madness and hemorrhoids were both punishments from Jehovah. A madman with a sore bottom would be evil indeed!

In Saxon times, from the 6th to the 11th centuries, treatments were rather basic and it was thought a good thrashing with a dolphin-hide whip was all that was needed to get rid of the bad spirits.

The First Asylums

Medieval treatments were no more enlightened than those from ancient times. One of the better-known asylums was Bethlem Hospital in London, often called "Bedlam." Founded in 1247, it originally cared for the poor, but over time it took in those considered "mad." The methods of treating the mentally ill in medieval times were harsh. By denying the sufferers mental stimulus, it was believed they would regain their equilibrium and become calm. As a result, they would be confined in dark, airless cells, tightly bound so as not to hurt themselves or their fellows. Whips and chains would enforce compliance. This may well have been influenced by the thoughts of Cornelius Celsus, a Roman writing in the 1st century CE, who recommended locking victims in isolated dark cells where they were alternatively flogged, starved, given laxatives, and locked in fetters to scare them back to mental health. His success rate was probably not that high.

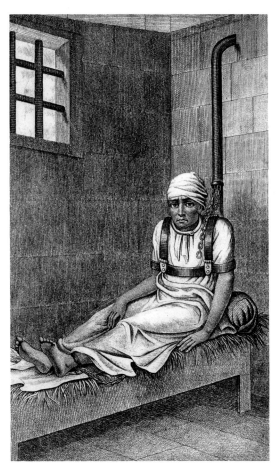

By Shakespeare's time (in ca. 1600), a derivative of this hospital's name had led to the word "bedlam" entering the English vernacular. Madness was also called the "English disease" and stock Shakespearean characters such as Hamlet and King Lear

RIGHT **James Norris spent at least ten years shackled to the wall in Bethlem Hospital. Concerned parliamentarians had him released in 1815 but he died two weeks later.**

may have been inspired by the dramatist's visit to Bethlem. Cures were simple and based on superstition. Borage and hellebore could be consumed, and roasted mice eaten in one gulp were seen as curatives. Leeching, vomiting, and beating were also popular remedies.

Asylums such as Bethlem were a must-see event on a day out. At the main entrance were two statues holding donation jars, and for a modest sum the public could have a great day out being entertained by the mentally ill. The public was allowed to wander at will, except to the basement where the real hard cases were kept, and take in the sights. The inmates would seek donations by rattling their chains and banging on their doors before singing ditties or capering around. The most entertaining patients were managed by warders, who summoned an audience like hawkers at a fairground.

In France, the first official asylums were pioneered by Louis XIV (1638–1715), at a time when madness was associated with political dissent; 6,000 suspect individuals were rounded up and confined in Paris's General Hospital during the 1660s.

BELOW **Visiting Bethlem Hospital was a popular pastime for wealthy and poor alike. The entrance fees lined the pockets of the warders rather than improving conditions for the mentally ill.**

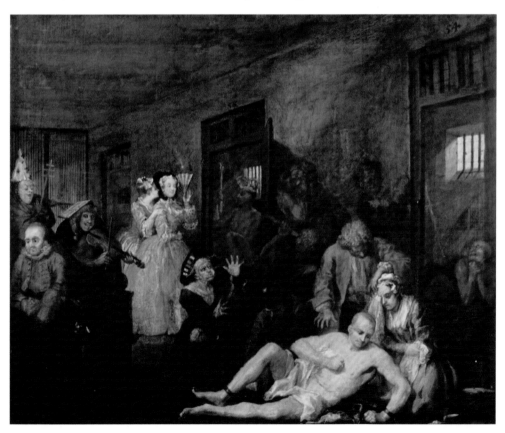

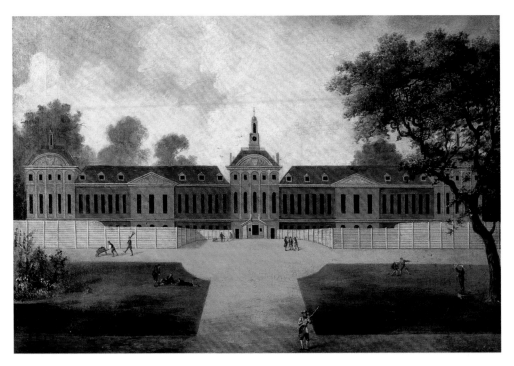

WORKHOUSES AND ASYLUMS

ABOVE **The proud classical exterior of Bethlem belied the chaos and suffering of patients within.**

In English society, many of the down and out ended up in workhouses. These became common throughout England when unemployment caused by the end of the Napoleonic wars (1815) and farm enclosures rose dramatically. Initially these dire institutions were almost as bad as prisons. In 1834 the Poor Law Amendment Act stipulated that a section of any poorhouse should be set aside for the mentally ill; this would be called the "Imbeciles' block." There were no treatments for the mentally ill, and conditions in workhouses were abominable, with inmates being routinely abused and living in unsanitary conditions.

However, if classified as insane, the inmates would be moved to privately run asylums and these were even worse. Political correctness was an unknown quality in those days and these houses were known as "madhouses." Like most privately run facilities, the driving motivation behind the formation of these houses was profit. Management tried to keep the mentally ill as cheaply as possible and with as little trouble as possible.

Management strategies included a wide variety of mechanical and physical constraints. Inmates would be packed into squalid, overcrowded cells or, if they were lucky, bare individual cells. It was believed that fresh air was a curative for mental "manias," so windows weren't glazed or covered, leading to a perpetual chill in the cells. Chains, cages, and leather straps were all employed to subdue the victims and the straitjacket, also known as the strait-waistcoat, was used to pinion violent or hyperactive inmates.

The York Lunatic Asylum opened in 1777 and was notorious for its shocking treatment of the mentally ill. Thirteen women were confined in a room 12 feet by 8 (3.7 by 2.4 meters). In another room were ten women chained by either an arm or a leg to the wall with only a blanket for covering. One inmate in Bethlem, James Norris, had been chained in a dingy subterranean cell for about a decade. Inmates were disciplined by floggings, cudgeling, and even rape.

Sane people were often wrongfully committed for political or legal reasons. Alexander Cruden was seized in 1753 and incarcerated in Bethnal Green Asylum, London, on the instigation of a rival for a young woman's affections. Decoyed to the madhouse, he was captured and chained to a bedstead. The following day the unfortunate Mr. Cruden was given a dose of physic which caused dreadful diarrhea, although no chamber pot was supplied. After that he was put in a straitjacket. Gaining the trust of the attendants, he was able to escape after ten weeks and prove his sanity to the authorities.

BELOW **This portrait of an asylum from 1735 depicts the terrible conditions prevalent at the time.**

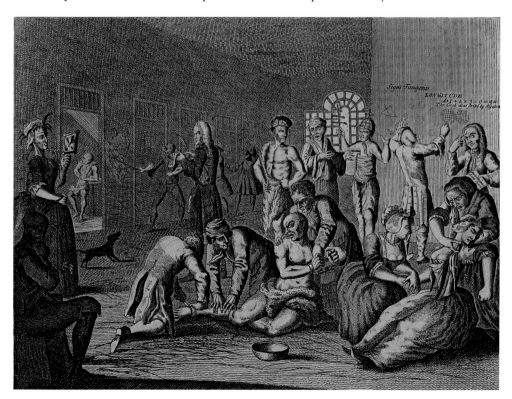

The author and journalist Daniel Defoe (1660–1731) campaigned for the rights of women who had been sectioned at the behest of their philandering husbands, and whose spouses had then seized the poor women's children and assets.

BLISTERING

Blistering was a particularly unpleasant treatment and had no beneficial outcomes whatsoever. It did have many negative effects though, including patients becoming obsessed with their genitalia. As insane people are often tormented mentally, it was supposed that it was good to make them suffer physically, in order to take their minds off their troubles. Blistering was well suited to this purpose. Blisters were raised with plasters smeared with a preparation of Spanish fly, a highly irritating and potentially lethal substance made when the European beetle *Lytta vesicatoria* is dried and ground into powder. The resulting concoction is a powerful, blistering irritant that can be absorbed through the skin or any mucous membranes. As well as causing nasty blisters, it has a diverse range of horrible side effects. It damages any tissue in which it comes into contact, and as it is excreted through urine, a heavy dose can lead to an acute inflammation of the entire urinary tract, which is termed urethritis. The tube along which urine is passed from the bladder to the penis or the urethral opening becomes horribly inflamed and painful. This makes urinating an incredible painful experience, and one of the main symptoms is blood in semen and urine. The bacterial infection can be so severe that it leads to the death of the sufferer. Another reported side effect, seemingly at odds with urethritis, was a rampant, insatiable erect penis. Patients became obsessed with their genitalia for obvious reasons.

The main reason that inmates were so tightly controlled with arm restraints and straitjackets was because of the fear of masturbation. The book *Onania: or the Heinous Sin of Self-Pollution (in Both Sexes)*, first published in 1730, ran to 15 editions. It gave a list of dire health outcomes resulting from this practice that included impotence, sterility, gonorrhea, skinny legs (at a time when healthy calves were the measure of a

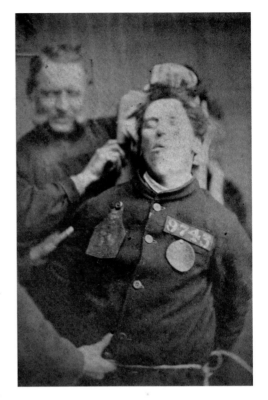

ABOVE **Restraint was the order of the day in most asylums. This inmate in Yorkshire, England, is being subdued by three warders in 1869.**

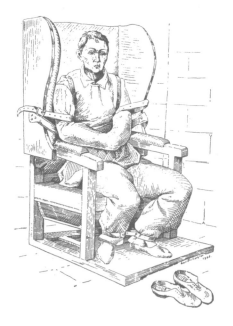

man), pasty complexion, fatigue, pimples, and weak jaws. Aaron Kaminski, whom many consider to have been Jack the Ripper, was committed when his "harmful indulgences" were blamed for his madness. It was believed that women who practiced masturbation would experience hysteria, spinal irritation, idiocy, depression, mania, and eventually death. Giveaway signs included loss of appetite and a shifty expression.

LEFT **Before the widespread use of sedatives, violent asylum patients could spend years in a straitjacket.**

RIGHT **A range of mental illnesses are depicted in this series of vignettes from 1858. Mental illness is no respecter of age, sex, or class.**

SCABIES

Inmates of asylums often died from skin infections and scabies due to poor treatment. Sickness was rife, with the ill forced to live in filthy straw, or on mattresses that would be hosed down once a week and then returned to the cells before they could dry out. Many visitors to Bethlem in the 18th and 19th centuries report scabies infections. Washing bedding in water was not enough to get rid of the mite.

Scabies is still a problem today in residential facilities. It is spread by the mite *Sarcoptes scabiei*. This tiny creature burrows into the top level of the skin and lays three eggs a day over a two-month period. The eggs hatch into larvae and travel back to the surface of the skin, leaving trails that can be clearly seen. The symptoms are guaranteed to send the mad madder; pimple-like irritations and burrows under the skin concentrate in skin folds around the knees, shoulder blades, elbows, genitals, and fingers. These create intense itchiness, especially at night when there are fewer distractions. The intense scratching often leads to sores breaking out that leak fluids and suppurate over time, sometimes leading to gangrene.

Elderly residents in asylums, or those with weakened immune systems, developed "crusted scabies," otherwise known as the "Norwegian itch." The skin becomes a thick, crusty hive of mites. Under the surface of the skin are living and reproducing insects as well the rotting corpses of dead parasites and their feces. This horrible leathery skin can cover the entire body except for the face and, even today, it is very difficult to treat as the crusty skin protects the mites.

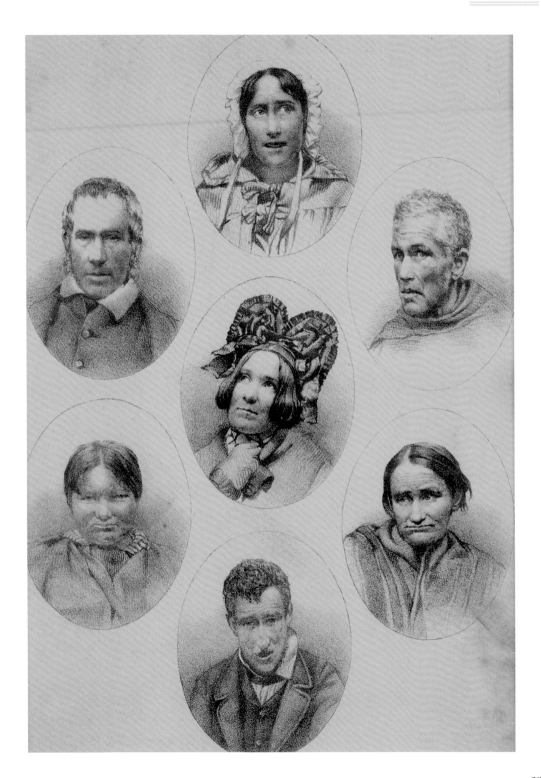

Chemical Restraint

By 1890, English asylums were catering to 54,000 patients; any earlier attempts to reform treatments were largely abandoned and restraint became the norm.

Chemical restraint became very popular and a wide range of sedatives was experimented with. Morphine, cannabis, amyl hydrate, hemlock, and ergot were all used either as a punishment or as a sedative. One of the most frequently used drugs was chloral hydrate, otherwise known as "knockout drops" or "Mickey Finns." Hyoscyamine was another frequently used drug with extremely unpleasant side effects. This was sourced from plants such as belladonna and mandrake and the side effects would be likely to make a person with mental issues feel even worse. They included blurred vision, bloating, constipation, drowsiness, dry mouth, excitability, headache, nausea, anxiety, muscle weakness, insomnia, rashes, hives, difficulty breathing, tightness in the chest, swelling of the lips, mouth, face or tongue, agitation, behavior changes, confusion, impotence, diarrhea, hallucinations, loss of consciousness, memory loss, mood changes, loss of taste, trouble urinating, and vomiting. Such a drug could easily be used as a threat to any troublesome patients.

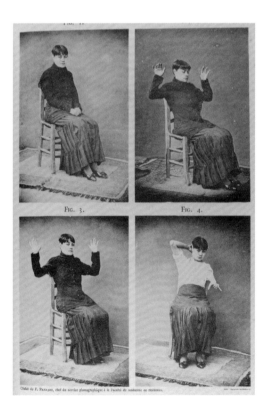

FIG. 3.   FIG. 4.

Female Hysteria

The Greeks believed that women were subject to hysteria. This was caused by the unfertilized womb moving around the body disturbing the four humors. Hippocrates (460–370 BCE) developed the theory that good health required a balance between four elements: blood, yellow bile, black bile, and phlegm. The recommended cure for hysterical women was permanent pregnancy. Hippocrates diagnosed this disease and noted that symptoms were fainting, seizures, pain in the chest, and mental derangement. He noted that it was particularly prevalent in virgins, widows, and spinsters, and recommended sexual intercourse as a cure.

LEFT **A patient in a cataleptic state experiences severe rigidity in the limbs. They may be locked in one position for hours.**

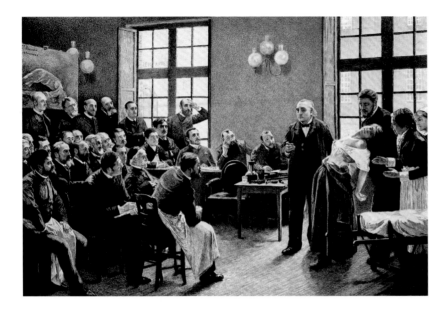

As late as the 19th century it was presumed that possession of a cervix caused an unstable emotional state among women, and they were particularly disposed towards either melancholia or hysteria. This was evidenced from puberty to menopause. Menopause was considered such a dangerous time for women that in the 1850s the English doctor Edward Tilt recommended that it should be delayed as long as possible by wearing underpants, taking cold showers, and becoming a vegetarian. What data he used to back these assertions is unknown. The good doctor did advise that feather beds and romantic novels could hasten menopause. He also advised that husbands should not have sex with their menopausal wives, and that aroused older women should be treated with ice-cold douches, enemas, and leeches applied to the labia, as these methods were sure to put a stop to any unseemly desires. Isaac Baker Brown performed innumerable clitoridectomies (female circumcisions) on his English patients in search of a cure; however, he was expelled from the Obstetrical Society in 1867 for malpractice.

ABOVE **French neurologist Jean-Martin Charcot demonstrating hysteria in a patient at the Pitié-Salpêtrière teaching hospital, Paris, 1887.**

In 1792, William Pargeter, an English pioneer in mental health, wrote in his book *Observations on Maniacal Disorders* that the main cause of madness in delicate-framed women was the inordinate consumption of tea.

"Female hysteria" was considered to be a common disorder among women but it is no longer recognized as a problem. The diagnosis of female hysteria was routine, particularly in 19th-century America and Europe. Women considered to be suffering from hysteria exhibited a wide array of symptoms, including faintness, insomnia, fluid retention, heaviness in the abdomen, muscle spasms, shortness of breath, irritability, loss of appetite for food or sex, and "a tendency to cause trouble." These symptoms can be caused by the menstrual cycle or the menopause, but any moodiness or dissatisfaction was attributed to the female condition.

The condition was widely debated in the medical literature of the Victorian era. In 1859 it was claimed that a quarter of all women suffered from hysteria. One American doctor recorded 75 pages of possible symptoms for the disorder, and still thought the list to be incomplete. According to his report, pretty much any ailment could fit the diagnosis for female hysteria. It was believed that the stresses associated with modern life made women more prone to nervous disorders, as well as faulty reproductive tracts. These tracts then had to be "exercised" in order to alleviate symptoms.

Once the mishmash of likely symptoms had been used to diagnose hysteria, the doctor would prescribe a course of weekly pelvic massages. During the treatment the doctor would manually stimulate the female's genitals until multiple "hysterical paroxysms" were accomplished. Hysterical paroxysms are, of course, orgasms. Few women practiced medicine during this era, so the opportunities for female doctors to give their patients orgasms was limited. Doctors

BELOW **Some "manifestations" of hysteria. Almost any expression or activity could be deemed as evidence of hysteria in women.**

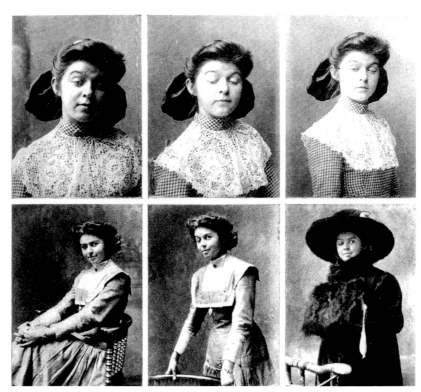

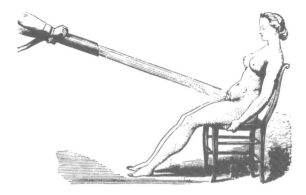

LEFT This French pelvic douche device was intended to suppress the female sexual appetite.

made a goodly profit from this procedure, since it represented repeat business and a low-risk procedure. Pelvic massages were used as a medical treatment on women right into the early 20th century.

Some doctors found it difficult to consistently give large numbers of women regular orgasms. In 1873, the first mechanical vibrator was developed and used at an asylum in France for the treatment of female hysteria. Initially these mechanical devices were only available to doctors for use in pelvic massages, but by the turn of the century, the spread of home electricity brought the vibrator to a broader market. The number of diagnoses of female hysteria sharply declined during the early 1900s, eliminating a profitable procedure for many doctors. Today it is no longer recognized as an illness.

MAD OR INSPIRED?

Joan of Arc's (1412–31) belief that she was in contact with a multiplicity of angels and saints led to her to inspire troops to eject the English from many of their possessions in her French homeland. They had been occupying huge swathes of territory throughout the Hundred Years' War (1337–1453) and it took Joan's divine intervention to begin the process of expelling them. She was able to convince the French authorities that God was on their side.

At the time of her trial she gave a detailed description of her visitations. Often beginning with bright lights, voices and visions gave her instructions that she was bound to follow. They began when she was 13 years old, and the first voice was that of Jesus telling her how to behave. It happened on a fast day in her father's garden and initially the Son of God's advice was to go to church and be a good girl. At other times, she heard a voice from her right, which was accompanied by bright light, and it repeated the messages three times, proving, in Joan's view, that it was an angel speaking. St. Michael than appeared and exhorted her to go to war and expel

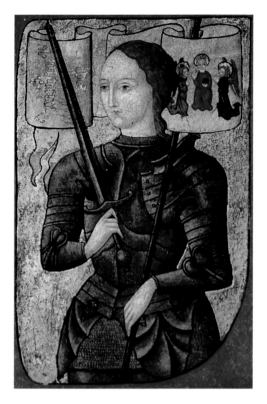

ABOVE **It is impossible to give an accurate diagnosis of Joan of Arc's mental condition. There is no doubt that she believed she heard voices.**

the English. Even as she stood trial and was committed to be burned at the stake, the voices continued to intrude on Joan's consciousness and direct her actions.

But was she mad or inspired? Joan of Arc is a textbook case of how hard it is to diagnose someone well after the event. There are at least ten different possible medical, psychological, or behavioral causes for her voices.

One possibility is that she suffered from Ménière's disease, an ear problem that can cause dizziness and auditory confusion that often presents as voices. Similarly, those suffering from tinnitus do not always hear a ringing sound but may hear voices, or hissing or buzzing noises. Another physical illness may have been a form of tuberculosis, which resulted in a tumor in the temporal region of her brain. Such a growth, which may have come from many other sources, can cause auditory hallucinations and visions.

She may have suffered from schizophrenia, which commonly causes voices and visions, and there is a possibility that she was bipolar or manic. Severe schizophrenic cases often feel that they cannot control their actions or are being manipulated by external forces. Psychotic tendencies have also been revealed. She was able to manipulate many people to a much greater degree than an unlettered farm girl might be expected to, and possibly the voices were a means to manipulate the Dauphin and "mad" King Charles.

Another possibility is that Joan hallucinated on a form of LSD. This often came about accidentally from eating contaminated grain. The fungus ergot grows on grains such as rye, barley, and wheat. Poor storage of grain, a common occurrence in the Middle Ages, allowed ergot to thrive. Ergot was known as "mad grain" and "drunken rye," because of the hallucinations it caused. The psychoactive ingredient in ergot is a form of LSD (lysergic acid diethylamide). LSD could possibly account for the "voices."

One expert expressed the view that Joan's hearing of voices was only one of several symptoms she exhibited. Due to malnutrition she suffered profound ill health (cachexia) including the absence of menstrual periods (amenorrhea); these are symptoms of those suffering from anorexia nervosa.

Then again, some sufferers of epilepsy have ecstatic visions and this may have been part of her makeup. Finally, it is possible that she had a classic case of dissociative identity disorder, otherwise known as multiple personality disorder. Often presenting in individuals who have been exposed to extreme violence, as occurred throughout huge swathes of the French countryside during the Hundred Years' War, people with this disorder protect themselves by adopting a number of personalities. It seems Joan would oscillate between great war leader, simple farm girl, divinely inspired prophetess, and crafty manipulator. The absence of menses is a common symptom of this disorder and it is believed that Joan did not experience regular periods.

A King Made of Glass

Joan of Arc was certainly not the only "mad" celebrity in France at the time. Charles VI of France (1368–1422) had begun as a wise and steady ruler but after several fevers his grasp of reality fell apart. His most persistent delusion was that he was made of glass and could be shattered at any time. He asked for steel rods to be sewn into his clothing to prevent this occurring. At times he thought he was a wolf, and would run through his palace corridors howling. At one stage he turned on several attendants while hunting and killed them. Holes were drilled in his skull and powdered pearl was poured in, but all to no avail, and he continued to be known as Charles the Mad.

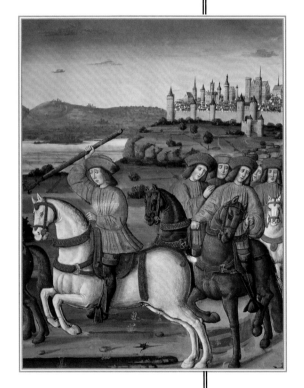

ABOVE **As a young man Charles VI possessed many knightly virtues, but as he became delusional he refused to ride a horse, fearing that he would fall and shatter into a thousand pieces.**

MAD KING GEORGE

The most famous deranged English royal was George III (1738–1820) who was on the English throne from 1760 to 1820. His first episode occurred in 1762 and blisters were applied to his forearms and he was bled. His initial symptoms—and these were repeated in his later attacks—were fevers, colds, coughs, and cramping. The "physics" obviously worked because he was much improved after several months.

When he was 50, George suffered another major attack. Although described as gout, this is unlikely as he had a very modern, healthy diet for the time, and enjoyed plentiful vegetables and water. It seems he had some sort of nervous breakdown combined with a fever and he would display signs of nervous

BELOW In James Gillray's cartoon, George III is satirized as the mad King of Brobdingnag, from Swift's *Gulliver's Travels*.

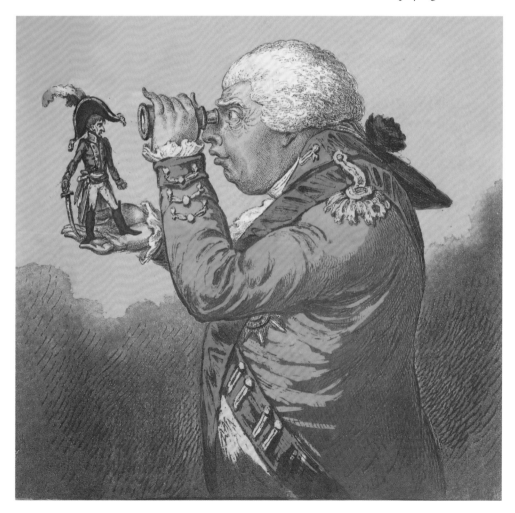

collapse in any stressful situation. His body seized up and rashes spread over his skin. He could not concentrate or read dispatches, let alone make a decision. His speech became intemperate and clear signs of mania were exhibited while he foamed at the mouth. At one stage he introduced himself to a tree, thinking it was the king of Prussia.

Eventually the only option was to restrain the king as he began writing non-sensical letters to foreign dignitaries, bestowed baronets on scullery maids, and became convinced that he had caused London to be flooded by the Thames. Dr. Willis was put in charge of his case and he separated the king from his family. The king became suicidal and would attack his attendants or swear at them and try to bite them. George was restrained whenever he misbehaved with a variety of straitjackets and purpose-built chairs. His legs were blistered (they suppurated for several weeks) and leeches were applied to his temples and chest.

Despite the often-controversial treatment, Dr. Willis perhaps did a good job and there were national celebrations when it was announced that the king had recovered in 1789. Such was the king's pleasure that Willis and his sons received pensions of £650 for the rest of their lives. However, more attacks followed and in 1801 Dr. Willis tried to cure George by staring at him.

The king's final episode began in 1810 when he fixated on a young duchess and his delusional state convinced him the two of them were having a torrid affair, despite the fact that by this time he was 72 years old and blind. George's manic state obviously rendered him unfit to rule and the Regency Act (1811) was passed allowing his son, George, Prince of Wales, to rule in his stead.

Many modern medical practitioners have tried to diagnose King George's madness. It has been suggested that in fact he was suffering from porphyria, which he inherited from his maternal or paternal ancestors. Symptoms include sensitive skin, colored urine, paranoia, hallucinations, and excessive hair. A sample of his hair was recently tested and it contained high levels of arsenic, maybe explaining some of his symptoms, especially his sore and stiff muscles. One symptom of porphyria is discolored urine, and George's attendants did report that his was blue. However, it appears that he was given medicine based on gentian and this also can turn urine blue.

It is more likely that George suffered from manic–depressive episodes brought on by a predisposition to bipolar disorder. From a study of his letters it has been determined that during his episodes, George became incredibly verbose and a single sentence could run for as many as 400 words. He would often repeat himself and he became more prolix. His never-ending ranting monologues are a classic sign of false euphoria during a manic phase of bipolar disorder. Such was his emotional state during these times that he would have fits, requiring his pages to sit on him to avoid self-harm.

LOBOTOMIES

The lobotomy is a type of neurosurgery, or surgery performed on the brain, known as psychosurgery. The justification for psychosurgery is that debilitating forms of mental illness can be treated by changing the way in which the brain functions. From the 1930s to the 1960s, doctors believed that by cutting the connections between the frontal lobes, or prefrontal cortex, and the rest of the brain, they could calm patients' emotions and stabilize their personalities without affecting with their intelligence and motor functions. The patient could then re-join society.

The prefrontal cortex performs a number of complex roles in the brain, commonly called "executive functions." (Creativity, expression, higher-level decision-making and planning, personality, reasoning, and socially acceptable behaviour are all governed by the executive functions.) The prefrontal cortex is linked to many other areas of the brain, including the thalamus, which receives and transmits sensory signals.

The brain is made up of two different types of matter: gray and white. Gray matter encompasses the neurons, or brain cells, as well as their blood vessels and extensions. White matter comprises the axons, or nerve fibers, that connect the areas of gray matter and carry messages between them through electrical impulses. A lobotomy

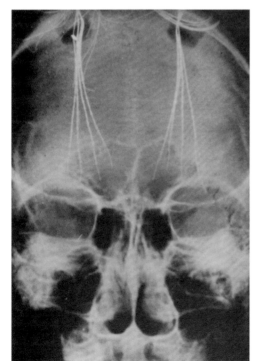

was intended to sever the white matter that linked different areas of gray matter. (An alternative name for lobotomy, leucotomy, means "white cutting" in Greek.)

The first recorded lobotomies were performed in 1935 by two Portuguese neurologists, Dr. António Egas Moniz and Dr. Almeida Lima. They initially drilled holes in the skull on either side of the prefrontal cortex and injected alcohol into the connecting fibers to destroy them. However, as could be expected, many complications ensued from this procedure,

LEFT **Modern medicine allows for electrodes to be implanted into the brains of those suffering from mental illness. These stimulate brain function rather than reducing it, as is the case with lobotomy.**

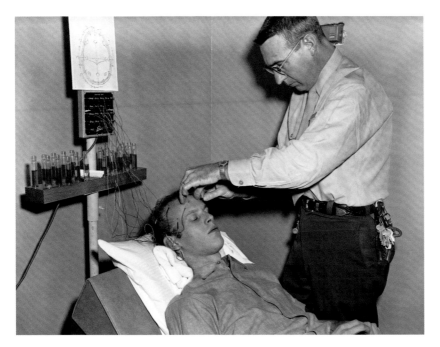

including damage to other parts of the brain. Moniz then designed a tool called a leucotome, which was inspired by an apple corer. After drilling holes in the skull, the doctor pressed on the back of the tool, which extended a loop of metal wire into the brain matter. He then would "core" the brain by twisting the handle, slicing off balls of white flesh before retracting the loop. The little detached pieces of brain matter were left inside, where they would be absorbed by the body over a period of time.

ABOVE **Dr. William Keating, the warden of California's Vacaville State Prison, believed that a lobotomy could cure criminality. This prisoner is being prepared for the procedure in 1961.**

There were other types of lobotomy more invasive than the Moniz method. J. G. Lyerly of Boston thought it was important to be able to see what he was doing, calling this "prudent visibility." While operating in the 1940s, he would remove large sections of the patient's skull that covered the frontal lobes, as if removing the cover from a fuse box. The lobes were then lifted or pushed aside to allow access to the white matter, which was cut with a small, sharp knife. He then cauterized the wound with a device like a soldering iron that seared the brain matter with much sizzling and crackling. The "lid" was then put back on and sutured back into place.

James Poppen, also of Boston, developed another type of open-topped lobotomy at the same time. He would drill very large holes in the top of the head and then use electrical devices to fry the offending white matter before sucking up the dead tissue with a surgical suction device.

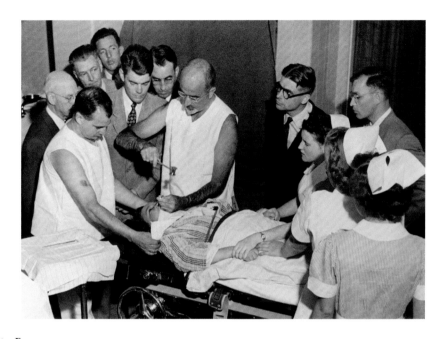

ABOVE **Dr. Walter Freeman was not averse to publicity. Here, he hammers an ice-pick-like instrument into a patient's frontal cortex.**

Freeman's Ice Pick Surgery

Dr. Walter Freeman (1895–1972) loved performing lobotomies on people—sick people, naughty people, even people in the wrong place at the wrong time. Families could get their troubled siblings, sons, or parents permanently sedated for as little as $200 a go. The beauty of the procedure was that it could be performed anywhere at any time. Trained at Yale University, Pennsylvania, he spread his message and technique throughout the United States.

During 1936 Freeman developed an improved version of earlier procedures that accessed the frontal lobe tissue via the patient's tear ducts. Known as the transorbital lobotomy, it was performed using a simple kitchen ice pick, later refined into a more efficient instrument called a leucotome, which was hammered through the thin layer of skull at the corner of each eye socket. Freeman would then swing the pick from side to side, damaging the frontal lobe. The process did not require the assistance of a qualified surgeon, took approximately ten minutes, and could be performed anywhere.

Freeman, it seems, invented this procedure with the best of intentions. He started out working as a neurologist at St. Elizabeth's Hospital in Washington, DC. This old mental institution with antiquated facilities had the capacity for 5,000 inmates. Each patient's upkeep was funded by state legislature at a meager $2 a day, which was to cover accommodation, food, treatment, medicine, and staff salaries. Freeman was shocked by the horrendous conditions in which the patients were living. The sight of the inmates' vacant stares and gibbering countenances filled him with fear and disgust. He therefore developed the transorbital lobotomy as a means to facilitate the return of the mentally-ill to return to the community.

Freeman's inspiration for the procedure came when he observed two chimpanzees that had had their entire frontal lobes removed—a lobectomy—in 1935. The animals had previously been nearly unmanageable, but the operation by John Fulton rendered them docile and compliant. Aware that invasive surgery often led to infections and deaths, he followed the 1937 work of an Italian, Amarro Fiamberti. The latter perforated the skull just above the eyeball in the orbital plate behind the eye sockets before injecting caustic solutions to destroy the white matter. This method of entry was called the "transorbital" approach. The problem was that the solutions often sunk down and destroyed much material in the spinal column and at the base of the brain.

Freeman and his associate James Watts decided to adopt the transorbital approach. The idea was that Watt the surgeon would do the surgery guided by Freeman. The two innovative gentlemen practiced on cadavers using a thin metal spike. The instruments that they were initially using were not strong enough and broke, leaving the tip within the corpses' skulls. Freeman rummaged through his cutlery draw at home and came up with an ice pick. He mounted a hammer-like handle on it that allowed it to be manipulated after it had been tapped through the skull. An improved version of this was called the "orbitoclast." After going through the top of the eye socket, Freeman could enter the brain just by tapping lightly on the orbitoclast with a hammer to break through the thin layer of bone. Then he twirled it to cut through the connective fibers. After pulling out the orbitoclast, the procedure was repeated on the other side. The transorbital lobotomy took ten minutes or less. Freeman first performed his transorbital lobotomy on Ellen Ionesco in 1946. She was described as "violently suicidal"; she was immediately cured.

ABOVE **A set of Watts–Freeman lobotomy instruments, ca. 1950. These simple devices were hammered into the brain and moved back and forth to sever vital nerve connections.**

A Man on a Mission

Freeman was obsessed with making a name for himself as a great innovator, and left a trail of wrecked lives behind him. He traveled thousands of miles across the United States to carry out demonstrations at asylums and hospitals. An instinctive showman, he sometimes ice-picked both eye sockets simultaneously, one with each hand. He had a buccaneering disregard for the usual medical formalities: he chewed gum while he operated and displayed impatience with what he called "all that germ crap,"

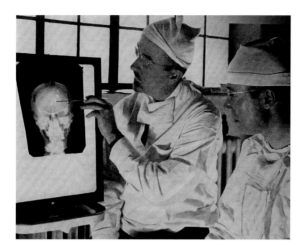

LEFT **Dr. Walter Freeman, left, and Dr. James W. Watts study an X-ray of a patient's brain before a psychosurgical operation.**

routinely failing to sterilize his hands or wear rubber gloves. Despite a 14 percent fatality rate, Freeman performed around 3,500 lobotomies in his lifetime. He once performed 25 lobotomies in a single day and developed a cavalier, messianic, or evangelical determination to spread the word and the procedure throughout the country. His championing of the procedure eventually included a traveling "lobotomobile," a customized van in which he demonstrated his technique to the press as well as to doctors at mental hospitals. Critics likened Freeman to an evangelist for the cause, while supporters claimed that getting a lobotomy was as safe and easy as getting a filling at the dentist's. Lobotomies cleared overcrowded hospitals, and unlike other psychiatric care, promised immediate results. Because the operation didn't require drilling through the skull, it could be done by rendering the patient unconscious via electroconvulsive shock. It could also be done by non-surgeons, which was handy since most mental hospitals didn't have operating rooms or surgeons on staff. Eventually, Freeman performed lobotomies as outpatient procedures in his office, in addition to doing them in mental hospitals and teaching other doctors how to do them.

Freeman enjoyed celebrity and cultivated certain journalists, propounding his theories and celebrating his "successes" in the mainstream media rather than the usual professional medical journals. Featuring on the front cover of many national dailies such as the *New York Times*, the positive headlines such as "Psychosurgery Cured Me" and "No Worse than Removing a Tooth" gave the operation a popular currency that no doubt made many take it up for their nearest and dearest.

Lobotomies Gone Wrong

In the United States, about 50,000 patients were lobotomized, most of them between 1949 and 1956. Dr. Freeman himself operated on at least 3,500 of them. He called lobotomies "soul surgery" and claimed that they could be used to treat not only schizophrenia, but also depression, chronic pain, and other mental and physical conditions. Freeman, and other doctors who performed lobotomies, believed that they could relieve suffering. In some cases, they did.

But in many they didn't. Three notorious cases come to mind. Howard Dully was a quiet, reserved boy who liked candy, reading, and collecting baseball cards. However, he did not like his domineering and emotionally distant stepmother and would seek to assert his independence by not cleaning his room and refusing household chores. Not unusual behavior for a 12-year-old boy. However, his stepmother had him lobotomized by Freeman in 1960. Unable to experience a normal life, he spent many years in institutions and perceived himself to be a freak.

At least Dully was conscious and had some internal awareness. Not so with Rosemary Kennedy, the sister of President John F. Kennedy. Beginning life as a shy and easygoing child, she became defiant and rebellious during puberty. Freeman was invited to perform a lobotomy on the 23-year-old woman and she became manageable—manageable like a vegetable. She lost the power of speech and could not control her bowels. She spent the rest of her life staring at the walls of mental institutions, finally dying at the age of 86.

Many other lobotomy patients had negative results. Anita McGee, who had suffered from postpartum depression, was lobotomized by Freeman in 1953. After the procedure, her daughter, Rebecca Welch, described her mother as "there but not there." McGee spent the rest of her life in institutions. Another case was Beulah Jones, who had been diagnosed with schizophrenia. She was lobotomized in the late 1940s. Her daughter, Janice-Jones Thomson, saw few positive outcomes from the procedure. Her behaviour did not improve—she just lost her long-term memory and the ability to read and write. Thomson also noted that her mother had lost her higher intellect.

Freeman's obsession with the procedure began to spiral out of control. He even invited his family to come and see him at work. His son Frank was invited to observe a lobotomy when he was 21 and vividly remembered hearing a little crack as the orbital plate fractured. Part of the drive to succeed came from Freeman's upbringing. Born in Philadelphia in 1895, he was driven from a young age to be exemplary, growing up in the long shadow cast by his grandfather, William Keen, an exceptional surgeon who was the first American to successfully remove a brain tumor. However, as the mounting stories of botched operations and needless deaths mounted, fewer surgeons were willing to use assembly-line lobotomies, he was ridiculed for his fanaticism, and the operation was banned in successive jurisdictions. He wife was an alcoholic, dying prematurely while Freeman engaged in a series of torrid affairs. He continued to perform lobotomies until 1967, when he was banned from operating after his last patient died from a brain hemorrhage following her third procedure. She had initially been lobotomized in 1946, then in 1956, and finally in 1967 when the ice pick tore a blood vessel. Freeman continued to visit his former patients and tout the success of the lobotomy procedure until he died of cancer in 1972.

11

SPANISH INFLUENZA

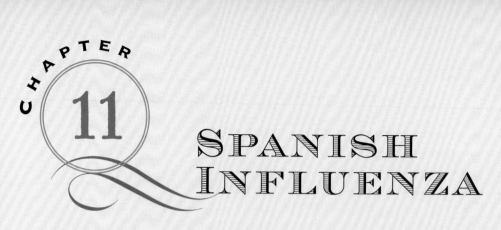

SPANISH INFLUENZA SWEPT THROUGH THE WORLD'S POPULATION between 1918 and 1919. Approximately 20 million deaths were recorded but the death toll may have been three times as high. Huge swathes of the developed world were affected, as were many Third World countries. It is estimated that 11 million people died in combat during World War I. The Spanish influenza was a much more efficient killing machine than all of the technological and industrial might of the world's great empires at the time.

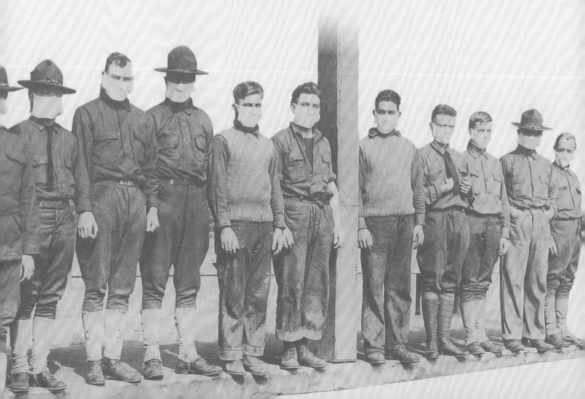

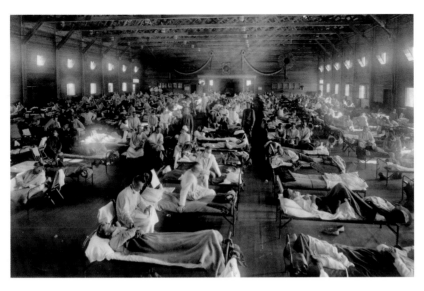

TRACKING DOWN THE SPANISH INFLUENZA

ABOVE The Spanish influenza ward at Camp Funston, Kansas, 1918. Army barracks were the ideal environment for the disease to spread.

The influenza virus has a long history of interaction with humans. It is a classic crowd disease and requires a particular density of humans to ensure that it thrives. The pathogen most likely crossed the animal–human barrier when pigs were first domesticated in the Near East approximately 15,000 years ago and in China 10,000 years ago.

Some strains can visit a population and cause barely more than a sniffle but others cause much more damage. The latter are lethal because even if immunity is built up to one virus, another strain will evolve rapidly and take our bodily defenses unprepared. The Spanish influenza was one of these; recent experiments show it had several unique features not seen in other strains that made it particularly deadly.

The flu virus experiences minor genetic shifts in its surface proteins two or three times each decade. These minor shifts allow the immunological response of humans to rapidly counter the new defenses and limit mortality. However, it is estimated that twice each century, or every 60 years or so, there is a major shift in the genetic makeup of the influenza virus that turns it into an immunological stranger to the existing population, allowing it to run rampant. The pandemic years 1833 and 1889 resulted from these genetic shifts, as did 1918, when the Spanish influenza struck.

After decades of searching, the preserved body of a young woman killed in the pandemic was exhumed from her tomb in the permafrost in Brevig, North Alaska. The microbiologist Johan Hultin had dug up some of the victims here in 1951. The virus had killed 72 out of 80 of the inhabitants of this tiny outpost, but Hultin could not obtain a sample of the virus. He returned in 1992 and this time enough slices of the young woman's lung could be collected to allow the extraction of the genetic material needed to work out the genome of the Spanish flu. Hultin finally succeeded in finding out why the virus, known as H1N1, was so deadly.

Researchers in a maximum biosafety facility at Canada's National Microbiology Laboratory reconstructed a fully-functioning virus and infected macaque monkeys to ascertain the strain's impact. The results were shocking. Within 24 hours of exposure to the virus symptoms appeared and the ensuing destruction of lung tissue was so extensive that, if the animals had not been put out of their misery, they would have literally drowned in their own blood. An earlier study using mice had described similar results. They also bore a striking resemblance to those described in human patients at the time the virus was at its most lethal.

A Lethal Strain

Why was this strain of influenza virus so lethal? Twenty million deaths were recorded in Western countries but other estimates range up to between 50 and 100 million casualties, 3 to 5 percent of the world's population at the time, and at least 500 million people were infected. The death rate was so high because the victims' own bodies turned on them. It was not the virus that directly caused the damage to the lungs—it was the body's own response to infection. Immune system proteins that can damage infected tissue were found at much higher levels following H1N1 infection compared with other viral infections. In 2005 analysis at the University of Wisconsin at Madison revealed that a key component of the immune system, a gene called RIG-1, appeared to be involved. This gene restricts and controls immune responses, ensuring that they only attack invading pathogens. Levels of the protein produced by the gene were lower in tissue infected with the 1918 virus, suggesting that the virus had a method of switching off RIG-1, allowing immune defenses to run wild to attack the host's own cells, not the invading virus.

THE OVERACTIVE IMMUNE RESPONSE HAD MADE THE VICTIMS DROWN IN THEIR OWN MUCUS AND BLOOD AS THE LUNGS' CELL WALLS HAD BROKEN DOWN, AND THEY WERE FLOODED IN EDEMAS CAUSED BY MULTIPLE HEMORRHAGES.

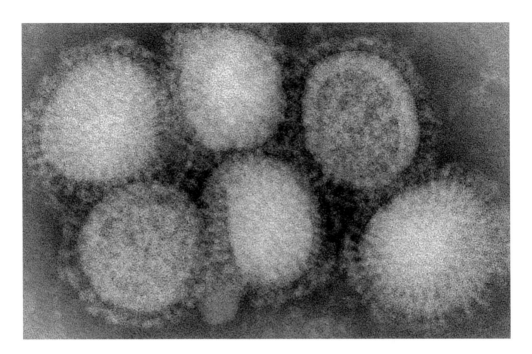

Most influenza outbreaks target the very young, the very old, or the very sick. The 1918 outbreak predominantly killed young adults. Their immune systems were so strong that they were most likely to cause damage as they went into overdrive. This condition, where there is an overreaction of the body's immune system, is otherwise termed a "cytokine storm." The strong immune reactions of young adults ravaged the body, whereas the weaker immune systems of children and middle-aged adults resulted in fewer deaths among those groups. Older people may have been given some protection by an earlier epidemic known as the "Russian flu" which struck 30 years earlier. The group that suffered most was pregnant women. The death rate among hospitalized women suffering from both complaints was up to 70 percent, and 26 percent lost their baby even if the mothers survived.

ABOVE Influenza virions. Every 60 years the flu virus undergoes a genetic shift. The Spanish flu was one of the most lethal strains in history.

Autopsies conducted on American soldiers struck down by the disease almost 100 years ago support these findings. The lungs are usually light and springy, filled with many air sacs. Some previous influenza victims might show some damage to their lungs, but the effects of the Spanish flu were much more drastic. The destroyed lungs were dense masses of flesh, soaked and heavy with a frothy, bloodstained fluid that had filled the entire chest cavity, allowing no oxygen to penetrate. The overactive immune response had made the victims drown in their own mucus and blood as the lungs' cell walls had broken down, and they were flooded in edemas caused by multiple hemorrhages.

Doctors at the time of the outbreak were shocked by the virulence of the disease. Many of the worst outbreaks occurred where thousands of fit young men were concentrated in American military barracks in preparation for shipping overseas to join the effort to end World War I. The robust appearance of the young men did not save them. The flu initially started out the same way as other coughs and colds with sore throats, a mild fever, and aches and pains. But then the virus's attack escalated and seemingly in an instant became life-threatening. Sufferers coughed bloody, foaming sputum as they gasped for breath. Their skin turned blue-black as mucus surged from the nose. The outpouring of blood was due to the virus causing hemorrhaging in the mucous membranes, stomach, intestines, and even the ears. This was often followed by death, sometimes less than 24 hours after the first symptoms appeared.

Initially the influenza's radical symptoms led to faulty diagnosis as dengue fever, cholera, or typhoid. Aiding this diagnosis was the fact that most influenzas have a mortality rate of 0.1 percent of those infected, while the Spanish strain killed up to 20 percent.

A SPANISH DISEASE?

It is not certain where the pandemic originated, but it is easy to explain why it was called the Spanish influenza. Though it also struck the French, British, American, and German forces mired in the trenches of World War I, their governments used censors to minimize early reports of the illness and understated the mortality statistics. The pandemic also struck in neutral Spain, where there were no such restrictions to reporting the devastating effects. King Alfonso was a high-profile victim and reporting gave the impression that Spain was particularly hard hit, therefore leading to the nickname of "Spanish flu." In Spain it was known as the "Naples soldier" after a "catchy" song with that title. Certain theories as to its origin have been proposed. Most agree that it originated somewhere behind the trenches on the Western Front in France. A major troop staging post and hospital complex was located at Étaples. This is a possible location from where the virus leaped from birds or pigs into its human hosts. Another theory postulates that the virus leaped from its original animal hosts in China, and was

Crazy Cures

Some believed that the Spanish flu could be cured by either eating raw onions, rinsing the mouth with lime water, inhaling turpentine fumes, or wearing cucumber slices on your shoes while carrying potatoes in your pockets. Alternatively you could inhale smoke from wet hay or breathe in chloroform vapors.

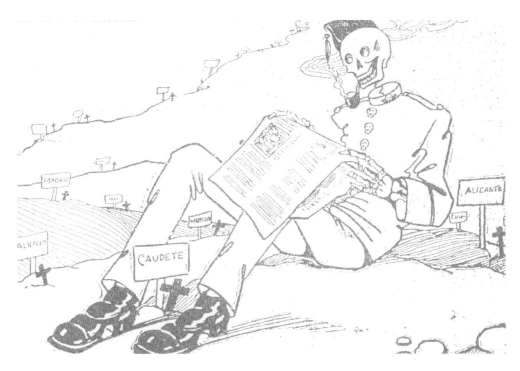

ABOVE **An artistic depiction of the "Naples soldier," a nickname for the Spanish flu.**

exported to the Western Front along with 96,000 Chinese coolies who labored behind the Allied front line.

The Institut Pasteur in France also attributes the first outbreak to China, but believes it first mutated to its uniquely deadly form in Boston, before being shipped out with Americans on troop transports to Europe. Others believe it may have originated in Kansas and, not to be outdone, the Austrians believe it originated near Salzburg in 1917. One radical theory even postulates that the virus arrived by meteorite before recombining its genes with an old virus, making a lethal new hybrid.

Whatever its origins, which will probably never be accurately traced, it was the peculiar circumstances of World War I that ensured it traveled around the world and infected up to half a billion people. The mass mobilizations characteristic of World War I saw hundreds of thousands of young men and women concentrated together in confined quarters, such as barracks, before being shipped all around the world in even more crowded circumstances aboard troop ships and trains. Some American towns were unaffected by the virus until military units paraded through the streets on their way to the European battlefields. As the soldiers were feted and kissed by loved ones, they infected the civilian population, setting off new pulses of the pandemic. Once at the front, the soldiers' immune systems were weakened by malnutrition, stress, and chemical attacks.

PANDEMIC

Once it got on its way, there was no stopping the deadly virus. Some have described the pandemic as the greatest medical holocaust in recorded history, and the first 24 weeks of the outbreak in early 1918 were particularly lethal. It is possible that in this 24-week period it killed more people than died during the "Pestilence" of the Middle Ages (see chapter 2: The Black Death).

As it cut its deadly swathe through humanity, almost no part of the inhabited globe was unaffected. The numbers are staggering: 17 million died in India; 23 million Japanese were infected and half a million died; 1.5 million died in Indonesia; in Tahiti almost 15 percent of the population expired in less than a month; and Samoa experienced a 22 percent mortality rate. Cold climates were not exempt and entire Inuit villages were destroyed or decimated, while Native Americans finally freed from the genocidal programs of earlier governments died like flies within their state-sponsored reservations. Canada lost 50,000 people, France 400,000, Brazil 300,000, Britain 250,000, and even African states such as Ethiopia were hit hard.

Poor decisions made in New Zealand allowed the pandemic to spread through the Pacific. No quarantine was initiated for ships arriving or leaving ports in that country, allowing the disease to be exported. This Kiwi-borne strain killed 8 percent of the population in Tonga, 16 percent in Nauru, and 5 percent of Fijians. These groups might have considered themselves fortunate compared to the disaster that struck New Zealand-controlled Western Samoa. Here, 30 percent of men, 22 percent of women, and 10 percent of children died, whereas American Samoa and French Caledonia imposed a blockade and suffered almost no casualties. Approximately 9,000 New Zealanders died.

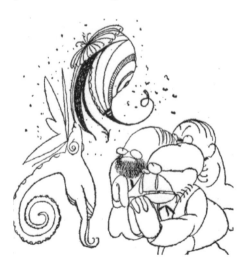

BELOW **A cartoon portraying biologists left powerless before the Spanish flu microbe.**

Australia was fortunate as the disease did not reach her shorelines before 1919, probably with returning servicemen, so many effective policies were initiated to limit its spread. Public venues such as schools, theaters, and churches were closed down once the flu was identified within a community. Facemasks were issued to all citizens, and once an individual was diagnosed their entire family would be placed in strict quarantine. Nevertheless, despite all these proactive measures, approximately 15,000 Australians aged between 15 and 35 perished, out of a population of 5 million.

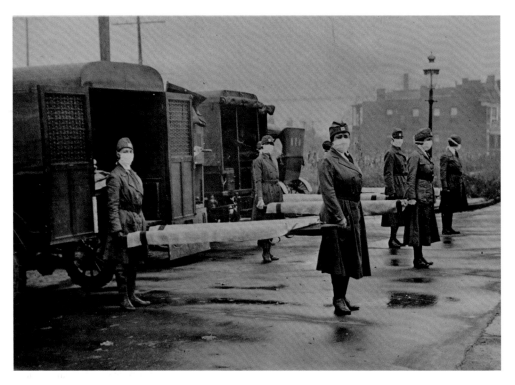

ABOVE The St. Louis Red
Cross Motor Corps was
mobilized to tackle the
October 1918 outbreak.

THE AMERICAN FLU

It could be appropriate to call the Spanish flu the American flu,
as the United States was particularly hit hard. At least 600,000
Americans died at home. The United States experienced 126,000 casualties in World
War I but of these only 53,000 died in combat: 73,000 died of disease and 43,000 of
these died from the flu—a massive casualty list.

Having recently brought in successful measures to counter yellow fever, the
medical establishment was shocked to find itself faced by an epidemic that it could
not contain. Naval nurse Josie Brown spoke of her experiences:

> *The morgues were packed almost to the ceiling with bodies stacked one on top*
> *of another. The morticians worked day and night. You could never turn around*
> *without seeing a big red truck loaded with caskets for the train station so bodies*
> *could be sent home. We didn't have time to treat them. We didn't take*
> *temperatures; we didn't even have time to take blood pressure.*

—JOSIE BROWN, NURSE

The U.S. Navy was uniquely well placed to see the effects of Spanish influenza as it crisscrossed the globe. The battle cruiser USS *Pittsburgh* was docked in Rio de Janeiro when two ships arrived from Lisbon and Dakar. Both reported cases of the flu but no attempt was made to quarantine the vessels by the Rio authorities. Within six days, hundreds of cases of the disease were reported in the city, while by the seventh day the *Pittsburgh* had a few cases. The next day the American naval ship had 33 sick sailors and the following day 92 cases had made their appearance on board. Hospitals onshore were full and not enough coffins could be supplied. By the eleventh day the flagship reported 418 casualties and most of the onboard medical staff were incapacitated. Cases peaked at over 600 and such were the conditions on board that the cruiser could not set out from port to patrol as ordered. Sailors had to lie on deck, no matter what the weather was like, due to overcrowding in the quarters, while "Ashore people died like flies, and many lay in the streets for two or three days waiting interment, even a hole in the corner of a trench." A report from the Admiralty demonstrated how troopships continued to transport soldiers to Europe despite the flu:

In fitting out transport medical departments, no expense was spared to make them as near to being real hospitals as possible. Each ship was fitted with a surgeons' examining room, dispensary, a laboratory, dental office, dressing room, operating room, special treatment room, sick bay, and isolation ward. In addition to these, several dispensaries and dressing stations were established throughout the ship for minor cases, which the troop surgeons utilized for those patients not requiring sick bay treatment.

The Spanish Influenza Epidemic taxed the resources of the transport medical departments to the utmost. Although every effort was made to eliminate sick troops at the gangway, it was inevitable that large numbers of incipient cases were taken on board, and naturally the crowded berthing spaces favored contagion.

As an example, during the September 1918, trip of the [transport, USS] George Washington, although 450 cases and suspects were landed before sailing, on the second day out there were 550 new cases on the sick list. Entire troop spaces were converted into hospitals. Strict regulations in regard to spraying noses and throats twice daily and the continual wearing of gauze coverings over the mouth and nose, except when eating, were rigidly enforced. The soldiers were kept in the open air as much as possible, while boxing bouts, band concerts and other amusements on deck were conducted to keep up morale. The result was gratifying and the epidemic was soon under control.

—*A History of the Transport Service; Adventures And Experiences of United States Transports and Cruisers In The World War*, Albert Gleaves, 1921

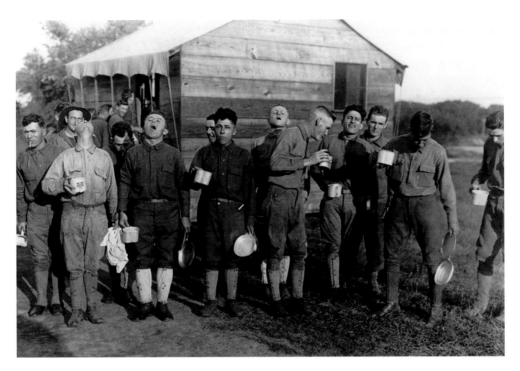

THE FIRST WAVE

Like the rest of the world, the United States was hit by three waves of influenza. The first recorded patient of the first wave was a company cook called Albert Gitchell, who reported to the camp doctor with flu-like symptoms on March 11, 1918. He was based in Fort Riley, Kansas, a training camp packed full of 26,000 recruits. Two hours later another soldier reported sick and by the end of the week 522 of Fort Riley's troops were laid up. Eventually 1,127 soldiers fell ill, and 46 died when pneumonia resulting from the influenza overwhelmed their lungs.

ABOVE One of the less than effective suggested preventatives for the Spanish flu was to gargle with salt water, as these soldiers in New Jersey have been instructed to do.

Other military encampments followed suit: California, Florida, Virginia, Alabama, South Carolina, and Georgia all saw outbreaks among the densely packed young soldiers. The Ford Motor Company in Detroit, Michigan, almost had to close when 1,000 workers fell ill.

The soldiers from Fort Riley carried the virus with them across the Atlantic. Landing in Brest and Saint-Nazaire in France, these towns too experienced an outbreak. It spread to the French army where it was named the "la grippe," before crossing the Channel and the Alps to infect the British Isles and Italy. The Royal Navy reported 10,313 cases and had to suspend operations.

The disease spread across the world and thousands died in the first manifestation of the "three-day fever," but it was merely seen as an inconvenience in sociopolitical terms. By the start of August 1918 it had died out. Authorities breathed a sigh of relief and continued with the serious business of killing each other with bombs, bullets, and bayonets.

THE SECOND WAVE

By the end of August 1918 a much more lethal version of the virus had arrived simultaneously in Freetown, Brest, and Boston. On August 15, 1918, Freetown, a port on the coast of Sierra Leone in West Africa, received HMS *Mantua*. Aboard this ship 200 sailors had a mild case of the flu, but five days later 500 out of 600 dockworkers had been struck by a far more lethal strain. Soon almost the entire population had been infected and mortality rates were far exceeding the first wave. The dock laborers were incapacitated, so the ships that put into Freetown had to use their own crews as navvies. There they contracted the virus, reembarked on their ships, and spread the infection onto their own vessels and across the oceans. Hundreds were killed in Brest in northwest France.

BELOW By 1919 the authorities had learned their lesson. These soldiers marching through Seattle wear masks to prevent transmission.

Boston was the first American city to see a major outbreak in the second wave of 1918. It first broke out in Commonwealth Pier where thousands of GIs awaited shipping to the war. Hundreds were infected,

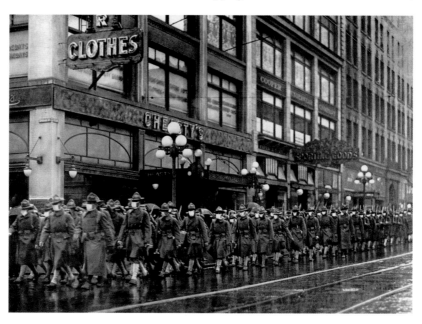

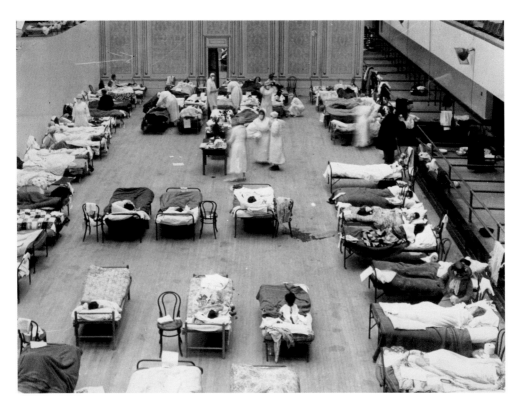

yet urgings that the place be quarantined were ignored. On September 3, 1918, Boston put on a patriotic parade entitled "Win the War for Freedom." One thousand soldiers from infected Commonwealth Pier marched in the parade and on that very same day the first civilian cases were reported. Plague-like events ensued, and even while it raged in Boston it also appeared in Portsmouth, New Hampshire; Newport, Rhode

ABOVE **Oakland Municipal Auditorium, California, 1918. Theaters and town halls became makeshift wards to cater for the high numbers of infected soldiers.**

Island; and Fort Devens, Massachusetts, an immense training camp packed with 45,000 troops. It was here that the disease really hit, alerting the authorities to the true nature of the new outbreak. Up to a hundred men would die each day. Colonel Victor C. Vaughan (1851–1929) was a veteran of many wars and was shocked by the scale of the outbreak, during which 7,000 men were crowded into a hospital built for 2,000. He saw how hundreds of fit and healthy young men were bought into the wards every day, resplendent in the uniform of their country. Soon their lips would turn blue, they would begin coughing blood, and in the morning their bodies were removed and stacked "about the morgue like cord wood."

NOT ONLY MEDICAL SERVICES BUT ALSO EMBALMERS AND UNDERTAKERS COULD NOT KEEP UP WITH THE WORKLOAD. BODIES ROTTED IN THE STREETS OR IN HOUSES ALONGSIDE FAMILY MEMBERS. SOMETIMES WHOLE FAMILIES SUCCUMBED, AND NEIGHBORS ONLY REALIZED WHEN THE STENCH LEAKED INTO ADJOINING PREMISES.

Doctors were shocked by what some termed a "vicious type of pneumonia." Two hours after admission mahogany-colored spots would appear above the cheekbones. Soon the discoloration would spread from the ears until it covered the whole face. Within two hours the young men died. Doctors were used to seeing one or two people die at a time but when the death toll reached 100 a day it was almost more than they could bear. Special trains were commissioned to haul away the dead but services were overwhelmed and not enough coffins were available.

The flu raged onward. In Massachusetts 85,000 were infected. Army bases were deemed to be such a hazard that the decision was made not to call up 142,000 men of the October draft. Philadelphia had its first case on September 12, 1918. On September 28, a crowd of 200,000 people met in the center of town for a war bonds drive and two days later 653 cases swamped the hospitals. So many medical practitioners were overseas at the front that the remaining doctors and nurses were overwhelmed. On October 10 in Philadelphia, 759 people died. Not only medical services but also embalmers and undertakers could not keep up with the workload. Bodies rotted in the streets or in houses alongside family members. Sometimes whole families succumbed, and neighbors only realized when the stench leaked into adjoining premises. Steam shovels dug trenches for mass graves, and prisoners were brought out in labor gangs to collect and dispose of corpses.

The previously untouched West Coast of the United States was also hit hard and San Francisco saw its first case on September 24, 1918. A young man, Edward Wagner, had recently moved there from Chicago and his house was quickly placed into quarantine. Masks were issued and public venues were closed down, but all to no avail. By October 19, thousands had been hospitalized and basic services had closed down. Garbage rotted on the streets, police were too sick to go on the beat, and fire stations had closed. On November 21, sirens finally announced the end of the epidemic, but this was only a temporary pause before another outbreak hit and by January 1919 there had been 50,000 reported cases and 3,500 deaths.

Densely populated metropolises were not the only American settlements to be infected. Brevig in North Alaska—where those samples of lung tissue were obtained in 1992—had a population of 80 people in 1918 and its nearest town was Nome,

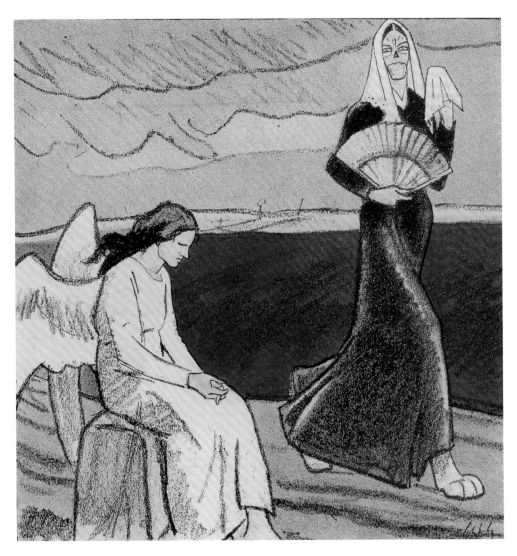

which could only be reached by dogsled. Two people visiting Brevig from Nome brought the virus with them. This remote indigenous population, which may well have survived smallpox and measles from the original European colonists, was decimated in a week and only seven people survived. Igloos were crammed with dead bodies. Some were eaten by starving sled dogs, while others comprised extended families with only one or two infants alive among their dead relatives. Dead and buried in the hard, frozen soil, one of these victims would eventually be disinterred and her lung tissue used to solve the mystery of why the Spanish flu was so deadly.

ABOVE **Just as peace seemed likely in Europe, the Spanish Flu seemed to bring a new horror. Here, the angel of peace is overtaken by the flu.**

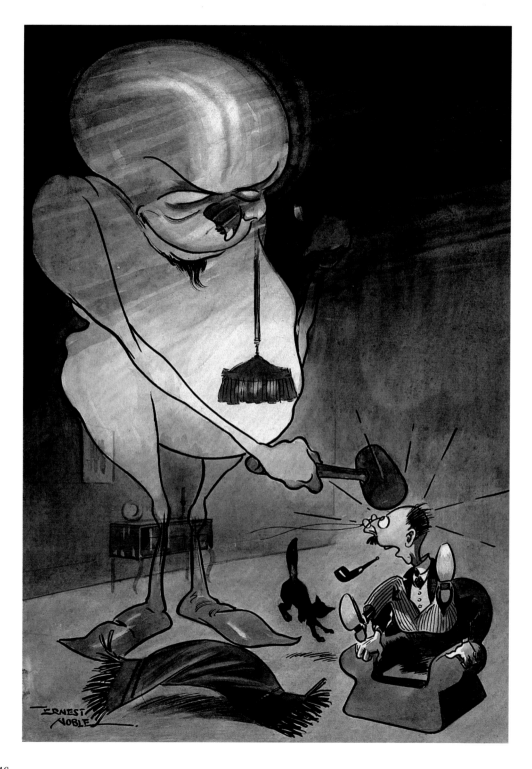

Rapid Decline

Just as a third wave seemed likely to overwhelm populations, the Spanish influenza stopped dead in its tracks and disappeared. Over the course of December 1918 and January 1919 around 3,000 Parisians died, while New York and San Francisco also lost thousands of people. But even before these events, overall numbers had begun declining. After the lethal second wave struck in late 1918, new cases dropped abruptly—almost to nothing after the peak in the second wave. In Philadelphia, for example, 4,597 people died in the week ending October 16, but by November 11, influenza had almost disappeared from the city.

One explanation for the rapid decline in the lethality of the disease is that doctors simply got better at preventing and treating the pneumonia that developed after the victims had contracted the virus. Another theory holds that the 1918 virus mutated extremely rapidly to a less lethal strain. This is a common occurrence with influenza viruses: There is a tendency for pathogenic viruses to become less lethal with time, as the hosts of more dangerous strains tend to die out. The most likely cause for its disappearance was that the disease had simply run out of people who were susceptible and could be infected. Whatever the reason, people were relieved to learn that the danger of infection to themselves and others had passed. In 1919, as news of the negotiations for the Treaty of Versailles became front-page news, signaling an end to the horrors of the war, it seems that people wanted to forget the war and the disease, seeing them both as part of the same horrible experience.

Influenza

The disease was first named *influenza* during 1781, from the Italian word for "influence." It was believed that celestial bodies such as planets, stars, moon, and sun were having a bad influence on affected individuals.

The most likely cause of the first outbreak of the flu was the domestication of pigs or fowl thousands of years ago. It is noticeable that even today, outbreaks in humans tend to be mirrored by outbreaks in another species.

LEFT **A monster representing an influenza virus hitting a man on the head as he sits in his chair. The flu could prove fatal for the very young and old. Adults were less likely to die from the disease.**

In its normal form influenza, colloquially known as "the flu," is a lot less deadly than the Spanish influenza. It is caused by a group of viruses that infect the respiratory tract. A highly variable set of viruses, they are constantly adapting and altering their forms, leading to a multiplicity of degrees of severity and a range of symptoms. In

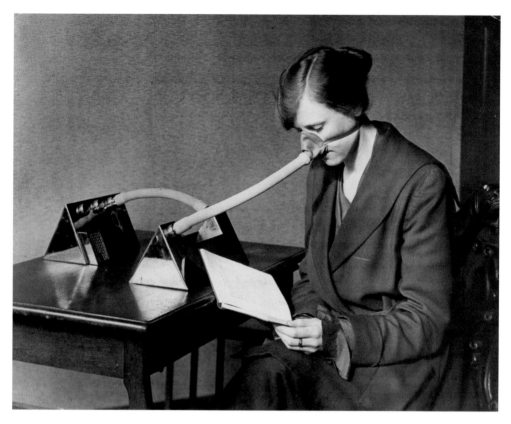

ABOVE **Artificial respirators were introduced as a preventative for the Spanish flu.**

temperate climates they usually occur between late fall and early spring, with between 5 and 20 percent of the population being infected. Mortality rates vary, but they are usually quite low, with the very young or very old being most likely to die. The mortality rate is usually about 0.01 percent and results from ensuing pneumonia. However, the flu is a major killer because so many catch it each year that even this low mortality rate leads to thousands or millions of deaths.

Influenza is mainly spread when infected people cough or sneeze, releasing small droplets of mucus that contain the virus. These are breathed into the respiratory tract of people around them. Additionally, an infected person can cough or sneeze on their own hands, and then contaminate objects which are subsequently touched by others who convey the virus to their mouth. The virus can live in the air for up to an hour, can survive on hard surfaces for up to eight hours, and on hands for up to five minutes. Infected carriers can shed the virus well before symptoms become apparent. It is generally believed that young children are the greatest spreaders of influenza, because they generate more viruses in their respiratory tract and are less likely to practice good hygiene.

There are two types of influenza viruses that cause serious disease in humans: types A and B. A third type, influenza C, causes a mild common-cold-like illness. Both influenza A and influenza B cause outbreaks and epidemics. Type A is usually responsible for pandemics. Like all viruses they survive by invading cells, where they replicate before bursting out from the corrupted cell to infect more cells. It appears that the A type was the original historical infection that arose in water birds such as ducks. The A type evolved within its new human hosts into the B type, which is now only found in humans.

The type A viruses are the most lethal and were responsible for the 1957 Asian flu pandemic, which killed several million people including 70,000 Americans, as well as the Hong Kong flu of 1968, which also killed at least a million people. Birds remain the most dangerous vector and some can carry up to 22 strains in their intestines without showing symptoms.

Bird Flu and Swine Flu

Both of these diseases are evidence that the influenza virus is continuing to cross from animals into humans. Bird flu (also known as avian flu) is the most dangerous to humans. In 2009, human swine flu was identified in the United States and named H1N1. It is a highly contagious variant, but thankfully it is rarely lethal in human or pig populations. Avian flu, H5N1, is an entirely different proposition. It seems that wild birds infected domesticated fowl in Asia before the illness jumped the species divide and infected its first human victim in 1997. Since then, 60% of those infected have died. Fortunately, human-to-human transmission is rare with H5N1 and most victims are those who work with commercial poultry. It is absolutely lethal to domesticated fowl and large numbers have been wiped out in Asia.

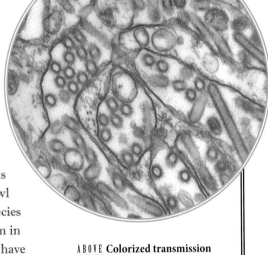

ABOVE **Colorized transmission electron micrograph of avian influenza A H5N1. It poses a small threat to humankind at present but there is no telling what the future could bring.**

FURTHER READING

Arnold, Catherine. *Necropolis: London and Its Dead*. London, Simon & Schuster, 2007.

Dobson, Mary. *Disease: The Extraordinary Stories Behind History's Deadliest Killers*. London, Quercus, 2008.

Gordon, Richard. T*he Alarming History of Medicine: Amusing Anecdotes from Hippocrates to Heart Transplants*. New York, St. Martin's Press, 1994.

Haeger, Knut (ed. and trans.). *The Illustrated History of Surgery*. Second edn, London, Routledge 2000.

Halliday, Stephen. *Newgate: London's Prototype of Hell*. Stroud, Gloucestershire, UK, The History Press, 2012.

Hollingham, Richard. *Blood and Guts: A History of Surgery*. London, BBC Books, 2008.

Karlen, Arno. *Plague's Progress: A Social History of Man and Disease*. London, Phoenix Books, 1996.

Lifton, Robert Jay. *The Nazi Doctors: Medical Killing and the Psychology of Genocide*. New York, Basic Books, 1986.

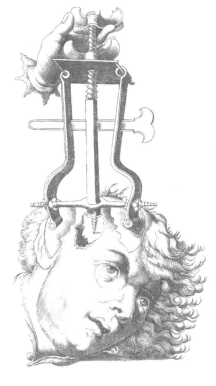

Schott, Ian, and Youngson, Robert. *Bad Medicine: True Stories of Weird Medicine and Dangerous Doctors*. London, Running Press, 2012.

Sugg, Robert. *Mummies, Cannibals and Vampires: The History of Corpse Medicine*. Abingdon, Oxfordshire, UK, Routledge, 2011.

Talty, Stephan. *The Illustrious Dead: The Terrifying Story of how Typhus Killed Napoleon's Greatest Army*. Victoria, British Columbia, Canada, Crown, 2009.

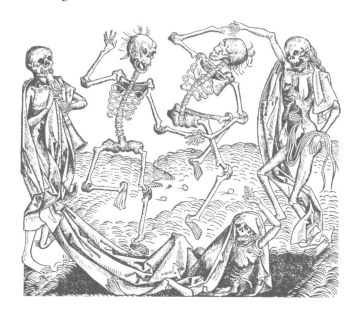

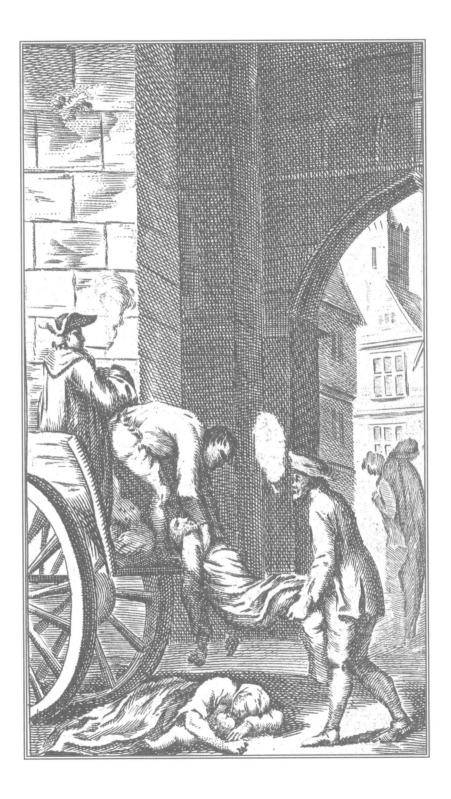

INDEX

Page numbers in **bold** refer to captions.

A

Abbott, Gilbert 92–3

accoucheurs 97

African trypanosomiasis 154

Agnolo di Tura 59

AIDS 68, 119, 123

Akbar the Great 203

Albert, Prince Consort 197

Alexander the Great 196–7

Alexander I of Russia 148

Alfonso XIII of Spain 236

ambulances 80

amputations 76–80

Amussat, Jean Zuléma 88

Anchises 30

anesthetics 90–4

Anson, Sir George 33

antiseptics 99, 100

Asclepius 89

Ashurbanipal 176

Asiatic cholera 153–4

Aspinall, George 205

asthma 17

asylums 211–15

Aurelia 89

avian flu 249

B

bacteria 7

baldness 17

Barbados leg 166–7

barbers 22

bathing 44

Báthory, Elizabeth 18

Batman, John 66–7

Becket, Thomas, Archbishop of Canterbury 44

bed rest 15–16

beriberi 204

Bethlem Hospital, London 211–12, 214, 216

bipolar disorder 210, 222, 225

bird flu 249

Black Assize, Oxford, UK 145–6

Black Death 36–53
  cures and preventatives 53–6
  disposal of dead 58–9
  flagellants 62–3
  Jewish persecutions 60–2
  plague today 63

black rats 43

bladder stones see stones

blaines 53

blistering 215

blood, uses of 18–20

bloodletting 13–14, 56

Boccaccio, Giovanni 38–40

body lice 139, 140–3

body parts, uses of 18–20

body snatchers 27

Boghurst, Dr. William 51–2, 54

Bolnest, Edward 19

botfly 70, 155

Brinkley, John R. 83

Broad Street Pump 190–2

Brontë, Emily 113

Brown, Isaac Baker 219

Brown, Josie 239

buboes 47, 52–3

bubonic plague 9, 36, 38–40, 45–7, 51–3

Buddha 89

Byron, Lord George 113

C

"cadaveric theory" 101

Caesar, Julius 89

Caligula, Emperor 28

camp fever see typhus

cancer 17, 20

carbolic acid 100, 101

carbuncles 51–2

Caroline of Bavaria 14

Cartier, Jacques 34

Casanova, Giacomo 72

caseous necrosis 114, 121

castration 83–5

cataracts 20

caudles 94

cautery knives 77

Celsus, Aulus Cornelius 87, 211

cesarean sections 89–90

chancres 67

Charcot, Jean-Martin **219**

Charles Borromeo, St. **43**

Charles II of England 16, 72, 117

Charles VI of France 223

Charles V, Holy Roman Emperor 28, 145

Chauliac, Guy de 35

chemical restraint 218

chicken pox 123, 137

childbirth 20
  cesarean section 89–90
  childbed fever 94–101

chloral hydrate 218

chloroform 81

cholera 8, 10, 100, 154, 185–94

Chopin, Frédéric 113

chronic diseases 9

Churchill, Frederick 93–4

Churchill, Sir Winston 67

Civiale, Jean 88

Claudius, Emperor 28

Clayton disinfectors **159**

Cleopatra 173

Clovis, King of the Franks 117

common cold 8, 20

condoms 72–3

constipation 17

consumption see tuberculosis

contraception 20

Cook, Captain James 35

cooties see body lice

Cortés, Hernán 134, 135, 136

cosmetics 18

cowpox 123, 130

Cox, Harold R. 151

crabs 71
  see also body lice

Crapper, Thomas 193

crowd diseases 10–11

Cruden, Alexander 214–15

Cuitláhuac 134

Culpeper, Nicholas 31

cytokine storms 235

D

dandruff 17

DDT 151, 163, 174

Defoe, Daniel 215

dengue fever 155, 162–3

dentistry 21–7

depression 210

Dickens, Charles 113

Digby, Sir Kenelm 21

Dionysus 89

Dioscorides, Pedanius 118

disassociation 210

dissociative identity disorder 223

Dostoyevsky, Fyodor 113

Dover's Powders 31

Drake, Sir Francis 203

Dully, Howard 231

dysentery 202–5

E

Ebola 9

Edward the Confessor 117

Eguía, Francisco de 134

electroshock therapy 209

elephantiasis 10, 164–8

Elizabeth I of England 25, 132

epilepsy 16, 17, 18, 19, 20, 21, 209, 223

ether 92

eunuchs 81, 83–5

Everett, Dr. Joseph 183

F

Fauchard, Pierre 23

feces

and disease *see* cholera; dysentery; typhoid; worms

medicines from 16–18

female circumcision 219

female hysteria 218–20

Ferdinand II of Aragon 145

Fiamberti, Amarro 229

fistulas 87

Flagellants 62–3

Flagg, Josiah 27

"flap" amputations 80

fleas 43, 44

Forde, Dr. Robert Michael 182

Fracastoro, Girolamo 184

Francis of Assisi, St. 110

Freeman, Dr. Walter 228

Fries, Lorenz 28

Frost, Eben 92

Fukuye, General Shimpei 204, 205

Fulton, John 229

G

Galen 118

gallstones 20

Gama, Vasco da 33, **154**

genital warts 8, 68

Geoffroy, M. 18

George III of England 224–5

Gitchell, Albert 241

gonorrhea 69

Goodyear, Charles 73

Gordon, Alexander 98

gout 28–31

graybacks
see body lice

Greeks, ancient 11, 21, 68, 79, 110, 128, 173, 209

Greenwood, John 27

Gustavus Adolphus of Sweden 146

H

Habsburg lip 28

Hansen's disease *see* leprosy

Hatshepsut, Queen 166

Hayward, Dr. George 93

Hazard, Isabella 188

head lice 71

hemorrhagic smallpox 127

Henry V of England 203

heritage diseases 9

hernias 35

herpes 68

Hippocrates 21, 30, 96, 110, 168, 173, 218

Holmes, Lt-Gen E. B. 205

Holmes, Dr. Wendell 99–101

Homer 30, 110

hospital fever *see* typhus

Hultin, Johan 233–4

Hunter, John 86

hygiene

medieval 44

Neanderthal 10

hyoscyamine 218

hysteria 218–20

I

influenza 8, 10, 136, 137, 247–9

bird flu 249

Spanish influenza 232–47

swine flu 249

inoculations 11, 100

intelligent design 37

Isabella I of Spain 44, 145

J

jail fever *see* typhus

Jamestown, Virginia 197

jaundice 17

Jenks, Rowland 145–6

Jenner, Edward 130

Jews, persecution of 60–2

jiggers 70

Joan of Arc 221–3

John, King of England 203

John of Burgundy 56

John of Gaddesden 20

Jones, Beulah 231

Justinian, Emperor 47

K

Kaminski, Aaron 216

Keats, John 113

Keen, William 231

Kehrer, Adolf 90

Kennedy, Rosemary 231

Kent, Countess of 17

Kerckhove, Dr. de 149–50

kidney stones *see* stones

"king's cure" 117

Koch, Robert 190, 199

Komyo, Empress 104

Kutuzov, Marshal 150

L

Laennec, René Théophile
Hyacinthe 121

Larrey, Dominique-Jean
80, 148

laudanum 94

Laveran, Charles Louis
Alphonse 169

lazar houses 107

lead poisoning 28

leeches 14

leishmaniasis 176–7

Leopold I of
Belgium 88

leprosy 9, 102–7, 154

Lettsom, John
Coakley 14

Lewis, Sarah 190–2

lice 71, 139, 140–3

ligatures 75, 79

Lillicrap, Peter 54

Lima, Dr. Almeida 226

Lind, Scott James 34

Lindow Man 206

Lister, Joseph 100, 101

Liston, Robert
90–2, 93–4

lithotrite 88

Livingstone,
David 179

lobotomies 226–31

Louis IX of France 69

Louis XIV of France
212

Louis XV of France
132

Louis I of Spain 132

LSD 222

Luther, Martin 97

Lyerly, J. G. 227, 229

M

McGee, Anita 231

macrophages 112–14

Magellan, Ferdinand 33

malaria 8–9, 137, 154,
168–74, 204

malignant smallpox 127

Mallon, Mary (Typhoid
Mary) 198–200

Manson, Patrick 167–8

Mary II of England 132

masturbation 215–16

mawworm 207

Maximillian II,
Emperor 145

measles
11, 122, 132–3, 137

medieval hygiene 44

Meigs, Charles 97

memorial portraiture
195

Ménière's disease 222

mental illness 208–25
   lobotomies 226–31

Mentuhotep II 166

mercury 64, 69

"Mickey Finns" 218

microfilariae 8

midwives 94–5

miliary tuberculosis
114, 121

Minos, King 72

modified smallpox 127

Mohan, Alice 93

Moniz, Dr. António
Egas 226

monkey implants 81–3

Montezuma II 134

Morton, William
92, 93

mosquitoes 8–9, 10, 155
   see also dengue fever;
   elephantiasis; malaria;
   yellow fever

Motolinía, Toribio de
Benavente 134–5

multiple personality
disorder 223

mumps 20

N

Napoleon
52, 147–51, 158, 203

Neanderthals 10

Nei Ching 173

Neisseria gonorrhoeae 69

Nelmes, Sarah 130

Nero, Emperor 28

Nicasius of Reims, St.
129

Norris, James 211, 214

Norwegian itch 216

Numa Pompilius 89

O

obsessive compulsive
disorder (OCD) 210

Onchocerca volvulus 177

opium 31, 209

Orford, Horace Walpole,
4th Earl 168

Ötzi the Iceman 30

P

Paganini, Niccolò 113

Papua New Guinea 154

Paré, Ambroise 77–9

Pargeter, William 219

Pasteur, Louis 100, 130

Pediculus humanus
corporis 140–3

pelvic massage 220–1

penicillin 67, 69, 154,
175–6

Pensacola, Florida 161

pentamidine 183

Pepys, Samuel 60, 88

Percie, George 197

Peter II, Tsar of Russia 132

Petit, Jean Louis 79

Philadelphia 159–60

Philip I of France 117

Phillips, Mrs. 73

Phipps, James 130

photography,
postmortem 195

phthisis see tuberculosis

"pinta" 175

Pires, Tomé 166

Pitt, William, the Elder
28–30

Pizarro, Francisco 136

plague see Black Death

Plato 209

pleurisy 17

Pliny the Elder 99

pneumonic plague 9, 37,
40–1, 47, 63

Poe, Edgar Allen 113

Poppen, James 227, 229

population dips 49

porphyria 225

postmortem
photography 195

Pott's disease
109–10, 115

pubic lice 71

puerperal fever 94–101

Q

quinine 174, 204

R

Rabel, Dr. 79

rabies 8, 10

Ramses V 128

Ramsey, William 207

Rays, Marquis de 154

Rejuvenation by Grafting 81–3

resurrectionists 27

Rickettsia prowazekii 138, 139, 140, 143, 144

"Ring Around the Rosie" 40–1

river blindness 177–8

Robert of Avesbury, Sir 62–3

Robert the Pious 117

Romans, ancient 11, 28, 68, 79, 99, 118, 128

Ross, Ronald 174

roundworms 206

Rush, Benjamin 163

S

scabies 70, 216

scarificators **14**

schizophrenia 210, 222

Schröder, Johann 21

screw tourniquets 79

scrofula 117

scurvy 32–5

Secrets, Dr. Don Alexes 55

Semmelweis, Dr. Ignaz 96, 101

septicemic plague 37, 41–3

Shakespeare, William 211–12

Shelley, Mary 97

Shelley, Percy Bysshe 113

ship fever *see* typhus

skulls 19, 20, 21

slave trade 158, 163, 179–80, 182

sleeping sickness 179–83

smallpox 8, 10, 100, 122, 123–31, 132
and the New World 133–7

smegma 17

Snow, John 192

somatization disorder 210

Soper, George 199

Spanish fly 215

Spanish influenza 232–47

Spence, James 25–6

spinal tuberculosis *see* Pott's disease

spring knives 14

stethoscopes 121

Stevenson, Robert Louis 113

stones 86–8

Störck, Baron von 31

streptomycin 119

styptics 77–9

surgeons 75

swine flu 249

syphilis 6, 8, 26, 27, 65–7, 72, 175

T

"taking the waters" 31

Tertullian 118

Thirty Years' War (1618–48) 145–6

Thompson, George 199

Thompson, Sir Henry 88

Thomson, Janice-Jones 231

Thucydides 128

Tiberius, Emperor 28

Tilt, Edward 219

tinnitus 222

toilets **17**, 44, 193

"tooth keys" 23

"tooth worms" 21, 23

T'ou-Shen Niang Niang 129

Tourette's syndrome 210

tourniquets 79

transplants 86

trephination (trepanning) 74, 209

tsetse flies 179, 181, 183

tuberculosis 9, 10, 27, 102, 103, 108–21, 222

turpentine 79

typhoid 10, 196–201

typhus
8, 136, 137, 138–46
and Napoleon 147–51
World War I 151

U

urine 16–18, 99

V

vaccinations 11, 100, 130–1

vascular system **56**

Vaughan, Colonel Victor C. 243

venereal disease 64–73

Vernon, Admiral Edward 158

vibrators 221

Victoria, Queen 197

viruses 6–7

vitamin C 32, 34

Voronoff, Dr. Serge 81–3

W

Wagner, Edward 244

Wallenstein, Baron von 146

war fever *see* typhus

Warren, Charles Henry 199

Warren, Professor John C. 92

warts 20
see also genital warts

Welch, Rebecca 231

West Nile Virus 155

whipworm 206–7

whooping cough 8, 20

Widal test 198

Willis, Dr. 225

Winterbottom's sign 181

Winthrop, John 158

Woolsey, Commodore Melancthon 161

workhouses 213

World War I
Spanish influenza 237, 239–42
typhus 151

World War II: dysentery 203–5

worms 9, 206–7

Y

yaws 9, 175–6

yellow fever
8, 10, 154, 155, 156–61

"Yellow Jack" 158

Yersinia pestis 37, 44

Yonge, James 80

Z

Zika virus 155

PICTURE CREDITS

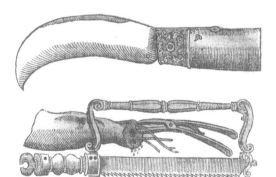

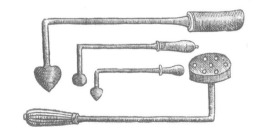